Health in France
1994-1998

Haut Comité de la Santé Publique
Ministère de l'Emploi et de la Solidarité
8, avenue de Ségur
75350 Paris 07 sp, France
Tel.: 01.40.56.79.80

Editions John Libbey Eurotext
127, avenue de la République
92120 Montrouge, France
Tel.: 01.46.73.06.60

All rights reserved. No part of this publication may be reproduced or transmitted in any form, or by any means, electronic or mechanical, including photocopy, recording, or any information storage or retrieval system, without permission in writing from the publisher.

© John Libbey Eurotext - Paris, 1999
© High Committee on Public Health
ISBN: 2-7420-0249-9

Ministry of Employment and Solidarity
High Committee on Public Health

Health in France
1994-1998

November 1998

High Committee on Public Health

President: the Minister of Employment and Solidarity

Ex-officio members: Director General for Health, Director of Hospitals, Director for Social Security, Director of the National Health Insurance Agency for Salaried Workers, Director of the National Institute for Health and Medical Research, Director of the National School of Public Health.

Members: Adrien Bedossa, Maryvonne Bitaud-Thépaut, Étienne Caniard, Jean-François Dodet, Pierre Ducimetière, Gilles Errieau, Bertrand Garros, Daniel Gautier, Michel Ghysel, François Grémy, Pierre Guillet, Albert Hirsch, Claude Huriet, Arnold Munnich, Guy Nicolas, Philippe-Jean Parquet, Jean-Daniel Rainhorn, Jean-Claude Sailly, Roland Sambuc, Maurice Tubiana.

Vice-president: Pierre Ducimetière

General rapporteur: Guy Nicolas

Secretary general: Joël Ménard, Director General for Health

Assistant secretary general: Geneviève Guérin

CONTENTS

	Foreword	7
	Introduction	9
Part one **Background to the health situation**	**Chapter one** Demographic, economic and social, political... considerations...	15
	Chapter two Public opinions and perceptions	35
Part two **Changes in health status**	**Chapter three** **Indicators of health status** General indicators Specific indicators	47 48 79
	Chapter four The determinants of health status Determinants linked to individual behaviour and the social environment Determinants related to work and the physical environment	145 147 185
	Chapter five Overview	211
Part three **A few organi- sational problems in the health system**	**Chapter six** Screening for female cancers in France	221
	Chapter seven Progress in emergency services	231
	Chapter eight Policy with regards to dependent elderly persons	245
	Chapter nine Comments	257
	Conclusion	267
	Acknowledgments	271
	Abbreviations, Lists of tables, figures, inserts and contents	273

Foreword

The French are in good health. In fact, they are healthier than ever before and we ought to be delighted. These statements are borne out by the present second report of the High Committee on Public Health: since 1991, average life expectancy has increased by almost one year and the mortality rate of those under sixty five years of age is constantly decreasing. Such undeniable progress puts our country amongst the most envied and privileged nations in terms of public health.

Our state of health continues to improve, thanks to the contributions made by a medical research effort of international stature, well-equipped hospitals, an adequate supply of physicians, and a consistently efficient social security system. The results are readily observable. The management of cardiovascular diseases and AIDS – to name but two examples – has improved and the number of deaths from these two causes is on the decline.

The High Committee also indicates some problem areas which ought not to be ignored. Firstly, greater emphasis is placed on cure rather than on prevention. It is the sick who dominate our health care system and not the hale and hearty who ask only that they remain so. This trend must be reversed, so that the system of patient management is actively involved in prevention instead of waiting for illness to strike.

In plain words, a whole change in outlook – a revolution – is required. Revolution is not too strong a word to use, given the apparently deeply ingrained attitudes that prevail. Only by overcoming such attitudes will we arrive at a more modern brand of medicine that will certainly be more effective and not necessarily more expensive. The user – and not the doctor – must be at the centre of the system with the doctor at his side.

The figures speak eloquently for other problems which remain to be solved. They show that heavy smoking, alcoholism, adolescent suicide and road accidents are the four main causes of excessive mortality in our country. All these scourges can be allayed by prevention, in other words, by informing the general public and providing health education, particularly to the young. This groundwork, based on persuasion and perhaps sanctions, must be undertaken as rapidly as possible if a few more additional precious years of life are to be attained.

Operations aimed at raising awareness should not make us forget the usefulness, equally preventive, of screening programmes for cancer (especially of the uterus, breast and colon) and hepatitis C which add to the load of suffering borne each year. Lastly, studies carried out under the aegis of the High Committee indicate that the French are paying increasing attention to environment-related diseases, *e.g.* those due to the presence of asbestos, and to the degradation in working conditions, such as persistent unemployment or job instability. Health involves a whole ensemble of factors.

With the publication of the present report and surveys published in the press based on data provided by the Ministry of Health, we are entering an era of health democracy in which discussions about public health priorities and the choices that they entail will no longer be the prerogative of a handful of experts but will be opened up to a wider audience of attentive citizens.

So, let the debate begin. May the States General for Health which are being organised in the different regions provide every one of us with a chance to become better informed, to understand, and to express our queries and opinions. I hope that I shall receive "health report forms" from all quarters which will serve as "complaints sheets" that we can all use as the basis in formulating our future healthcare system.

Bernard Kouchner
Secretary of State for Health

Introduction

The general report on "Health in France" was published by the High Committee on Public Health in 1994 and was an immediate success. For the first time, an analysis of the health of the French population was presented, based on the collective efforts of numerous experts, with a summary being given in the first part of the general report. First of all, it should be pointed out that this work was educational and instructive. Public health stands at the cross-roads of many disciplines and employs concepts which are not immediately obvious. Perhaps the most difficult idea to define is that of health itself! Is it as easy to say "the health of the population is improving" as "I'm currently in good health"? When speaking of the health of a group or population, reference is implicitly made to a particular health model: the latter might, for example, place its emphasis on the life-span of its members, or the very low incidence of observed deficiencies, or each individual's quality of life and personal development... or it might attempt to combine all these various attributes... One important result from such questioning is the realisation that the total resources mobilised by a population for health purposes (*i.e.* the health system) are not limited to those intended solely for "sick" individuals (*i.e.* the healthcare system), even if those who are ill form the most obvious and most ethically necessary part of any health system. Such questions were long regarded as theoretical and unimportant by a large part of the population, including the majority of healthcare professionals, as long as the resources committed by the community were affordable and did not seem to pose a threat to the very principles on which social protection operates, and especially the principle of solidarity. A few years ago, we reached the limit of what could be borne by the community, resources can no longer be stretched indefinitely, and it comes as no surprise that these questions are at the core of very pragmatic, topical discussions concerning the future of social protection and reform in the health system.

Once the declared objective of the health system is seen to be the fulfilment of the population's health requirements, the offer of healthcare – long considered an aim in itself – can then become the subject of regulation and unavoidable debate.

But we still have to be able to define the "health requirements" of the general population! Obviously, there is no absolute reference situation which could be used as the foundation in defining "requirements". At the most, all we can do is speak of a process or approach: this would be based on comparisons in time and space of all the observed aspects of the population's present health status and would lead to the formulation of what we consider to be "health problems". If we assume that the democratic process can go forward by determining the major problems for which targets must be set, it becomes evident that defining the health requirements of the general population is tantamount to working out a health policy. This form of procedure was described by the High Committee on Public Health (HCSP) in its December 1992 report, *"Stratégie pour une politique de santé" (Health policy strategy)* which demanded that a pluralistic, ambitious yet realistic approach be adopted that strove to be consistent whilst fully appreciating practical considerations and the need for feasibility.

Bearing this in mind, drawing up a periodic report on the state of the population's health means effectively analysing the progress so far made in defining, applying and evaluating health policy. Obviously, the HCSP 1994 report constituted an advance pronouncement in this respect. By showing that our country's state of health was in danger of deteriorating in spite of heavy expenditure on health, it signalled the need to make public health decisions – another way of expressing its wish for a structured health policy, a policy which even now has still to be worked out.

Most countries which are comparable to France, especially European countries, are confronted by similar problems, even if they differ widely in terms of individual health systems and the solutions they are trying to introduce. So it is not surprising that the drafting of health status reports is on each country's agenda : most reports are on a national scale, but some are regional, as in the case of Germany and Spain. The United Kingdom, Finland, Sweden, and Holland prepared at least one report of this type in the 1990s and adopted very similar points of view where their diverse acceptations of the concept of health was concerned.

At the present time, all the experts seem to agree on two essential points:
– the status of a population's health depends on many determinants and an understanding of such determinants is one of the objectives of biological, medical and health research. The determinants may be endogenous (inherited or acquired) or collective in scope – such as those affecting the environment, lifestyle, social interactions, etc. and, obviously, the status of medical techniques for prevention, treatment and rehabilitation. Health policy

can make a definite contribution to improving the health of the general population by acting on those determinants which are open to modification;

– the health system is not a closed operating system. Apart from its intrinsic determinants it does, in fact, largely depend on the general standard of living conditions as defined in demographic, economic, social and cultural terms. Thus, the status of the health system is also affected by the policies conducted in these domains.

Any analysis of the system which covered such a large number of interactions would necessarily be very complex. It would also be difficult to draw up a report on the status of the population's health that was not merely descriptive but additionally capable of playing an active role in structuring a health policy. Thus, a certain amount of diversification is being seen in the form and contents of reports in several countries with, for example, reports on specific topics being added to the main report issued every few years.

Since publishing the 1994 report, the High Committee has firmly opted for this approach. Whether at the particular request of the Minister for Health or via studies addressed to the National Health Conference and Parliament since 1996, the High Committee on Public Health has engaged in a detailed analysis of specific sectors of the health system and repeatedly requests that a coherent health policy be defined.

Under the final summary heading, *"Public Health must be given a free hand"*, the 1994 HCSP report stated that *"In spite of reservations and obstacles, it will still be possible for public health to make progress"*. The second part of the report directly supported this statement by indicating the route to be taken. A concerted consultation of health experts unprecedented in our country led to the identification of major health problems and determinants and the suggestion of indicators: this was subsequently completed by establishing relevant targets. Resulting from a co-operative effort by the DGS and HCSP, the consultation had a notable impact. Regional health Congresses used its proposals as the basis for establishing regional priorities and, in some cases, later regional health Programmes. The predominant determinants and health problems that had been identified were described in the HCSP report to the first national health Conference in 1996 and acted as the source for the latter's list of public health priorities submitted to Parliament.

Four to five years after the "Health in France" report was drafted, the HCSP felt that it would be appropriate to examine the current situation regarding the previously suggested indicators. Accordingly, the outlines of a "progress report" were sketched so that a few milestones could be marked out for an *a posteriori* evaluation of public health policy. At the end of its second mandate

Introduction

(1995-1998), and even though the resources at its disposal are limited, the High Committee on Public Health is delivering a report which should enliven the discussions opened up in the second part of the 1994 report. No attempt is made to compile an exhaustive set of statistics, the aim being rather to continue the instructive approach begun in 1994.

The second part of the 1994 report stated: *"It is not sufficient to put forward targets designed to minimize health problems. Conditions must also be arranged such that institutions and professionals may contribute to achieving targets, and such that individuals, families and communities may improve their health"*.

The plan of the present report is largely inspired by this comment. It seemed useful to give an outline in the first part of changes that have taken place in the health situation in France during the 1994-1998 period, given that a very important role is played by demographic, economic, social, political and institutional considerations. A further factor which must be taken into account consists of the general population's opinions and perceptions concerning the health system: the description of changes that have taken place in the latter between 1992 and 1997 is primarily based on the results from sample surveys carried out in these two years by CREDOC at the request of the HCSP.

Developments in health status are described in the second part, and variations in health indicators and determinants are successively tackled.

Lastly, the third part deals with three examples of problems encountered in organising the health system which, for the past few years, have been the subject of debate in France.

Pierre Ducimetière
Vice-President

PART ONE

Background to the health situation

CHAPTER ONE

Demographic, economic and social, political... considerations

Since publication of the first HCSP report, several different changes have occurred in France which have sometimes had a profound effect on the health situation. Hence, this first chapter is devoted to reviewing the changes that have taken place so as to facilitate the analysis of data presented below concerning the status of the health system and to put the data into more accurate perspective. Changes are viewed from four angles: (i) demographic, (ii) economic and social, (iii) political and institutional, and (iv) that of overall European health policy.

Demographic changes

Fertility and the birth rate have been recovering since 1995

Since the beginning of the 1990s, the French fertility rate has undergone fairly irregular changes (table 1). Although the "conjoncturel" fertility indicator remained steady at about 1.8 children per woman between 1985 and 1992, it took a sudden plunge in 1993 and 1994 to 1.65 children per woman. Starting from 1995, this indicator rose slightly but its 1997 level (1.71 children per woman) is still far removed from the value noted ten years ago.

Table 1 **"Conjoncturel" fertility indicator**
(births per 100 women)

	Births
1980	194.5
1985	181.4
1990	177.7
1993	165.4
1994	165.4
1995	170.2
1996	172.2
1997	171.0

Reading: 100 women who presented with 1997 fertility conditions at every age, throughout life, would give birth to 171 infants.
Source: INSEE, civil status statistics.

It is tempting to see these changes as a function of fluctuations in the economic cycle since the start of the decade. More specifically, there appears to be a correlation between variations in fertility and changes in the "morale" of individual households as measured by indicators used in economic surveys among couples. An age-based analysis confirms that fertility has registered shifts in behaviour arising out of certain economic conditions. Up until 1992, the stability of the global fertility indicator resulted from a drop in the fertility rate of those under 30 and an increase in the fertility rate of those over 30: both these changes have been regularly noted since the start of the 90s. In 1993 and 1994, the decrease in the fertility rate accelerated among the young while the over-30 fertility rate remained stagnant: both these trends contributed to a large drop in the global fertility rate. A renewal of long term trends – *i.e.* a drop in the under-30 fertility rate accompanied by a strong over-30 increase – accounts for the upswing observed in fertility starting from 1995 (table 2).

Table 2 **Fertility according to age**
(births per 100 women)

	Total	15-29-year-olds	30 and over
1980	194.5	141.8	52.7
1985	181.4	124.9	56.5
1990	177.7	110.7	67.0
1993	165.4	98.3	67.1
1994	165.4	96.2	69.2
1995	170.2	96.5	73.7
1996	172.2	95.2	77.0

Reading: 100 women who presented with 1996 fertility conditions at every age, throughout life, would give birth to 172.2 infants, including 95.2 among 15 to 29-year-olds and 77 among those 30 and over.
Source: INSEE, civil status statistics.

There have also been irregular changes in the number of births that result not only from variations in fertility but also in the number of women of child-bearing age. While approximately 800,000 children were born in 1980, the number of births in 1994 was only 711,000. Since 1995, it has fluctuated between 725,000 and 735,000, with the nadir in 1997 (table 3).

Table 3 **Number of births**

	Births (in thousands)
1980	762.4
1985	759.1
1990	743.7
1993	711.6
1994	711.0
1995	729.6
1996	735.3
1997	725.0

Source: INSEE, civil status statistics.

Marriages and divorces are on the increase

A pronounced drop in the annual number of marriages was recorded at the beginning of the 90s. A slight increase had been observed at the end of the 80s, with 287,000 marriages taking place in 1990. This figure decreased by 11% up until 1994 and 1995 when only 254,000 marriages were celebrated per year. However, 1996 saw a very marked increase, followed by a modest rise in 1997 when 285,000 marriages took place (table 4). This spectacular increase was probably partially due to fiscal measures that revoked the sometimes favourable income tax situation enjoyed by unmarried couples.

Table 4 **Number of marriages**

	Marriages (in thousands)
1980	287.1
1985	280.2
1990	271.4
1993	255.2
1994	253.7
1995	254.7
1996	280.6
1997	284.5

Source: INSEE, civil status statistics.

Part one Background to the health situation

Although a lasting inflexion in matrimonial behaviour has yet to be confirmed, the change in family structures since the beginning of the decade has been characterized by a continuing increase in the number of divorces (121,000 in 1995, i.e. 38.7 divorces per 100 marriages) and in the number of births outside of wedlock (39% of all births in 1996). These changes were accompanied by an increase in the number of both single-parent families (one family in eight, including one child in nine according to the 1990 census) and "reconstituted" families (consisting of a couple and at least one child from a previous union of one of the two adults) – it is difficult to estimate, but the number of the latter was put at 660,000 in 1990 (including 950,000 children). The concept of a family therefore bears less and less resemblance to a sole model of two married parents and their children.

Mortality continues to drop

There were 534,000 deaths in 1997. This figure corresponds to the annual mean for 1995 to 1997 and is slightly higher than the mean for the period 1990-1994 (table 5). However, these variations do not indicate any inflexion in long term mortality trends. While the gains in life expectancy slowed down in 1996 and 1997 because of influenza epidemics, age-adjusted mortality still shows a marked downward trend. In reality, the slight increase in the number of deaths since 1995 is due to the fact that the number of persons aged 65 and over in the general population is on the increase.

Table 5 **Number of deaths**

	Deaths (in thousands)
1980	526.2
1985	524.7
1990	521.5
1993	532.3
1994	520.0
1995	531.6
1996	536.8
1997	534.0

Source: INSEE, civil status statistics.

There was a dramatic drop in infantile mortality in 1995, with 4.9 deaths before the age of one year per thousand live births. However, in spite of a slight upswing, the infantile mortality rate noted in 1997 (5.1 ‰) is significantly lower than the 1994 level (5.9 ‰). In large measure, this striking decrease is the result of a drop in the number of "crib deaths".

The decline in general mortality has been accompanied by an increase in life expectancy (table 6). At birth, life expectancy has progressed by 1.5 years for men and 1.2 years for women since the start of the 90s, and now stands at 74.2 years for men and 82.1 years for women. More than half this gain is due to the decline in mortality after the age of 60. In 1996, a 60-year-old Frenchman could expect to live another 19.7 years and his female counterpart another 25 years.

Table 6 **Life expectancy according to sex and age**
(in years)

	Men		Women	
	at birth	at 60 years	at birth	at 60 years
1980	70.2	17.3	78.4	22.4
1985	71.3	17.9	79.4	23.0
1990	72.7	19.0	80.9	24.2
1993	73.3	19.4	81.4	24.6
1994	73.7	19.7	81.8	25.0
1995	73.9	19.7	81.9	24.9
1996	74.1	19.7	82.0	25.0
1997	74.2		82.1	

Source: INSEE, civil status statistics.

For the first time, the proportion of 20-64-year-olds in the population has decreased

The last few years have seen a regular increase in the proportion of persons 65 and over among the total population. In contrast, the proportion of those under 20 has diminished by almost two points since 1990. Up until now, the overall result of these two different trends did not affect intermediate age brackets and their share in the total population remained stable. However, a reversal occurred in 1996 when, for the first time, the percentage of 20-64-year-olds in the total population began to shrink, even though the decrease was very slight (table 7). Although largely symbolic, this trend made the consequences of ageing among the general population more readily visible.

Table 7 **Percentage distribution of population as a function of age**
(on January 1st)

	Under 20	20-64 years	65 and over	Total
1980	30.6	55.4	14.0	100.0
1985	29.2	58.0	12.8	100.0
1990	27.8	58.3	13.9	100.0
1995	26.1	58.9	15.0	100.0
1996	26.0	58.8	15.2	100.0
1997	25.9	58.7	15.4	100.0
1998	25.8	58.6	15.6	100.0

Source: INSEE, civil status statistics.

Part one Background to the health situation

Economic and social considerations

Economic growth has been slow

Even if 1993 was an exception in that it saw the most marked decline in activity (- 1.3%) since the end of the Second World War, it is still true to say that France has seen very modest economic growth since the start of the 90s, *i.e.* a mean of 1.2% per annum in constant francs. This actually represents half the potential growth rate of the French economy which has been evaluated at 2.3% per annum on the basis of full utilisation of production facilities and continuing trends in productivity.

The different components of the gross domestic product have undergone various changes (table 8). Growth in the main component, *i.e.* household consumption, has matched that in the economy as a whole (1.4% per annum on average), whereas investment has sharply declined (- 1% per annum). Foreign trade has made a positive contribution to growth with a significantly higher annual increase in exports (4.3%) than in imports (2.5%).

The latest available data provide a contrast with the general gloom which has characterized the 90s. Growth of 2.4% was recorded in 1997, with recovery starting in the second quarter and persisting throughout the remainder of the year. The annual growth rate was 3.2% in the fourth quarter, so that strong growth of about 3% can be expected.

Table 8 **Percentage growth and its principal components from 1991 to 1997**
(at 1980 prices)

	1991	1992	1993	1994	1995	1996	1997
Gross domestic product	+ 0.8	+ 1.2	- 1.3	+ 2.8	+ 2.1	+ 1.5	+ 2.4
Imports	+ 3.0	+ 1.2	- 3.5	+ 6.7	+ 5.1	+ 2.8	+ 6.6
Total resources & employ.	+ 1.3	+ 1.2	- 2.0	+ 3.6	+ 2.7	+ 1.8	+ 3.4
Household consumption	+ 1.4	+ 1.4	+ 0.2	+ 1.4	+ 1.7	+ 2.1	+ 0.9
Investment	+ 0.0	- 2.8	- 6.7	+ 1.3	+ 2.5	- 0.5	+ 0.2
Exports	+ 4.1	+ 2.6	- 0.4	+ 6.0	+ 6.3	+ 4.7	+ 11.3

Source: INSEE, social accounting.

Employment is stationary and unemployment rising fast

Between 1990 and 1996, total employment (self-employed and employees, including national service conscripts) declined by about 200,000 (table 9). Within the same period, the working population rose by 760,000 as a result of demographic factors and a continuing increase in levels of employment, mainly among women. The total number of unemployed rose by almost one million between 1990 and 1996. In 1996, unemployment affected 3,160,000 individuals, *i.e.* 12.4% of the potential working population. However, the 1997 upturn in growth led to considerable job creation (+ 130,000 over the entire year) and a fall in unemployment to only 12.1% of the potential working population by January 1998.

Table 9 **1990 to 1996 Labour Market**
(yearly average, in thousands of persons)

	1990	1991	1992	1993	1994	1995	1996
Active population	24,853	25,032	25,121	25,189	25,324	25,378	25,613
Employment	22,648	22,683	22,531	22,259	22,221	22,447	22,451
Unemployment	2,205	2,349	2.590	2,929	3,103	2,931	3,162

Source: INSEE, social accounting.

In the last few years, employment trends have been marked by an increase in atypical jobs such as those involving fixed term contracts, temporary posts, training courses, etc. In March 1997, these forms of employment represented almost 10% of salaried jobs compared with only 7% four years earlier. Part-time employment has also risen sharply. Almost 17% of those employed – and even 31% among women in gainful employment – held a part-time job in 1997. The rapid expansion in part-time employment is due to financial incentives designed to encourage its development that were introduced from 1992 onwards. However, part-time employment is increasingly seen as a stop-gap measure and almost 40% of part-time employees questioned by INSEE during the March 1997 employment survey indicated that they were looking for full-time work or wanted more work.

Lastly, the various categories of employees are not equally affected by unemployment. Unemployment tends to rise as the level of education drops: 17.4% of workers without any qualification or with only a primary leaving certificate are unemployed compared with 7% of those with a higher educational diploma. In terms of socioprofessional categories, the unemployment rate is three times lower amongst those in managerial posts (5.1%) than amongst blue collar workers (15.8%).

Part one Background to the health situation

Disparities in income have widened slightly since the mid-1980s

The transformations which have affected the operation of the labour-market since the mid-1980s resulted in a wider spread in salaries up until 1994 (figure 1). There has been a major increase in income from assets so that in spite of boosting mechanisms for social and fiscal redistribution (particularly by establishing minimum welfare benefits in 1988), inequalities in lifestyle have shown a minor increase (table 10).

The most recent data to become available seem to indicate that this trend towards wider disparities came to an end in 1994. The range of salaries and inequalities between men and women narrowed slightly, and surveys among households also supported the assumption that disparities in lifestyle had levelled off.

Figure 1 **Variation in the spread of salaries**

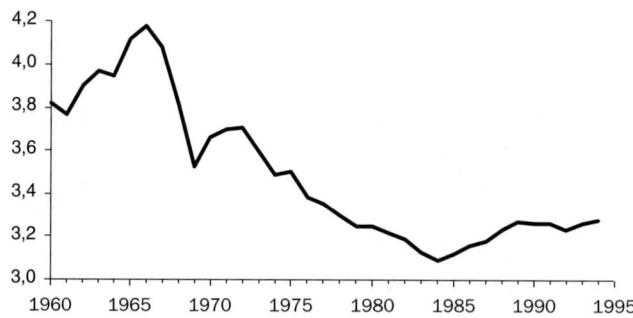

Reading: in 1960, the net salary separating the 10% best paid employees was 3.82 times higher than that separating the 10% least well paid employees.

Source: INSEE, annual declarations of social data.

Table 10 **Variation in lifestyle disparities**

	Inter-decile ratio
1984	3.81
1989	3.89
1994	4.01

Reading: the inter-decile ratio is the ratio of the lifestyle of the 10% most affluent households to the lifestyle of the 10% least affluent households. The ratio showed a regular increase between 1984 and 1994.

Source: INSEE, "Family budgets" survey.

Changes in the characteristics of poor households

The notion of poverty in households is complex and therefore difficult to define. One of the measurements used in its definition is relative and refers to the distribution of the entire set of incomes. Thus, households are considered "poor" when the available income per person[1] is half the level of income enjoyed by 50% of all households. According to this definition, the proportion of poor households remained stationary at about 10% between June 1984 and June 1994 (table 11). However, since there was an increase in the income level reached by 50% of households, the income of poor households in 1994 was higher than in 1984 in absolute terms.

Nevertheless, this global measurement of poverty masks important transformations that have affected the population of low-income households. As table 11 shows, poverty sharply declined among elderly households but rose in young households and single-parent families. The poverty of elderly households is related to low retirement benefits: it appears to have given way to households whose members are of working age and in which increased unemployment has been one of the major causes of poverty.

Table 11 **Percentage of poor households in 1984, 1989 and 1994**
(as a percentage)

	1984	1989	1994
According to the age of the person taken as reference			
Under 30 years	9.3	11.2	18.5
30-39 years	8.0	9.5	9.6
40-49 years	11.8	9.5	10.2
50-59 years	10.5	9.8	9.3
60-69 years	10.7	8.0	6.1
70-79 years	12.7	8.4	5.5
80 and over	13.8	11.9	11.6
According to household composition			
One person (60 and under)	8.3	9.0	11.9
One person (over 60)	11.0	9.2	7.6
Childless couples (60 and under)	4.5	4.3	5.7
Childless couples (over 60)	11.6	8.2	5.4
Couples with 1 child	6.4	5.9	7.1
Couples with 2 children	8.4	8.6	9.5
Couples with 3 or more children	22.6	21.0	19.7
Single-parent families	13.8	20.4	20.5
Other households	15.0	11.4	14.3
Total	10.4	9.6	9.9

Reading: in 1994, the income of 9.9% of households was below the poverty line, i.e. approximately 3 200 francs per month and per consumption unit. To determine a household's number of consumption units, the first adult is counted as 1, each subsequent adult as 0.7, and each child under 15 as 0.5.
Source: INSEE, "Family budgets" survey.

---

1. More exactly, per unit of consumption, i.e. counting the first adult as 1, each subsequent adult as 0.7, and each child under 15 as 0.5.

Thus, in households where the head of the household is unemployed, 39% have resources that are below the poverty level.

This brief account gives only a general idea of the diversity of situations covered by the term "poverty". A recently published, extensive INSEE study on poverty showed that while a quarter of households are at a disadvantage in terms of either living conditions (an accumulation of handicaps), or income, or even "subjective" (perceived) poverty, these three situations are found concurrently in only 1.7% of households. Hence, poor households can apparently be divided into three concentric circles: a "hard core" with a combination of difficult living conditions (about 2% of the population), low-income households (10%), and a collection of households (about 25%) expressing a high degree of dissatisfaction.

Political and institutional considerations

Stricter legislation governing biomedical ethics has been introduced

The following four laws were adopted by Parliament in July 1994 and equipped France with much more structured legislation dealing with biomedical ethics: the law of 1 July regarding the processing of named data for the purposes of health-related research, the law of 25 July concerning the protection of persons participating in biomedical research, and the laws of 29 July concerning respect for the human body, and the donation and utilisation of components and products of the human body as well as medically assisted procreation and prenatal diagnosis. Without going into the details of these very important texts which place France amongst those countries with the most enlightened legislation in this domain, a reminder should be given of their most essential principles.

Henceforth, the code of civil law clearly sets out the principles which govern the status of the human body, affirming the pre-eminence of the individual, prohibiting any affront to the dignity of the latter, and guaranteeing the respect for human life from the moment of conception. The laws also state that where the transfer and utilisation of human body components and products are concerned, the principles of prior consent, exemption from payment and anonymity must be applied. Commercial advertising is forbidden, though not information by the public authorities, and sanitary requirements must be met so as to protect the population.

Moreover, the law of 1 July 1994 is an adaptation of the law of 6 January 1978 concerning data processing and basic rights so as to cover certain aspects specific to medical research. It creates a balance between the freedom of the individual, respect for individual privacy and the value of aiding progress in medical research for the sake of the population's health. Thus, the law authorises the communication of medical data required in compiling files intended for health-oriented research, it permits departures from the rules of professional secrecy so as to allow the transmission of data derived from research projects authorized by the CNIL ("Commission Nationale de l'Informatique et Libertés" = National Commission on Data Processing and Basic Rights), and it provides for cases in which, for ethical reasons, individuals cannot be informed beforehand.

A reform in social protection is on the way

In common with several other reports, the 1994 HCSP report highlighted the need for far-reaching changes in the organisation of our health and social protection system. The reform which was introduced early in 1996 did, in fact, appreciably modify the organisation of the system. Up until a constitutional amendment was voted by Congress in February 1996, Parliament's prerogatives in health matters had been limited solely to government budgets: after the vote, Parliament was allowed to come to a decision on the entire budget for social protection. This development was later completed in April 1996 by three orders concerning respectively the organisation of social security, the control of medical healthcare costs, and the reform of public and private hospitalisation. Numerous points are covered in the three texts and, from the public health angle, it would be useful to place particular emphasis on two of these points.

Consideration of health priorities

The first point concerns those provisions which strengthen the link between health priorities and the allocation of resources. The orders effectively state that every year the finance bill submitted to Parliament by the Government must take into account health policy priorities and guidelines for therapeutic management put forward by the "Conférence nationale de santé" (National Health Congress). This authority has 78 members, including 38 representatives from the healthcare professions and institutions in public and private sectors, 26 representatives from regional congresses and 14 qualified persons. One of the prime aims of this congress is to analyse data concerning the health situation and the evolution of health requirements among the general population and to suggest the priorities which ought to be set in matters of public health policy and guidelines for healthcare management, given the advances made in preventive, diagnosis and therapeutic techniques. The finance bill formulated by the Government and submitted to Parliament is accompanied by the report drafted by the National Health Congress and also the report given to the National Congress by the High Committee on Public Health.

Agreements concerning targets and management subsequently finalised jointly by the Government and Branches of the National Health Insurance Agency, in line with the relevant appropriation bills, must mention the guidelines spanning several years of Government action in the area of public health and must define targets for improving the quality of service to users and targets related to the policy for social action and prevention. The conditions for implementation of these agreements are regularly examined by an independent monitoring committee which formulates and presents its opinion to Parliament. In addition, regional appropriations for hospital expenditures are fixed every year by taking into account public requirements and national or local priorities in terms of health policy with the aim of gradually reducing regional disparities in resources[2].

At the regional level, several provisions have also been made in reforming the health system so as to allow the emergence of regional health priorities and ensure that they are given effective consideration. A Regional Health Congress is initially set up with the role of establishing the region's public health priorities and putting forward proposals for improving the public's health status given all the medical, social, and medico-social resources available. The report of the Regional Congress is forwarded to the National Congress, the regional Agency for hospitalisation, the regional Union of Health Insurance Funds and the Union of physicians in private practice.

The regional Agencies for hospitalisation sign contracts setting out resources and targets with health care institutions. The contracts are of several years' duration and define quality and safety standards in health care and also the implementation of guidelines adopted by the Regional Health Congress. Additionally, the regional Agency for hospitalisation sends an annual progress report to the Regional Health Congress describing the actions taken by health care institutions that correspond to the health priorities that have been singled out by the Congress.

The regional Unions of Health Insurance Funds contribute to each individual Fund's implementation of health education and preventive measures needed for compliance with regionally determined public health priorities.

---

2. The HCSP drew up proposals in this area in the report *"Allocation régionale des ressources et réduction des inégalités de santé"* (Regional allocation of resources and reduction of health inequalities) by a working party presided over by J.-C. Sailly, 1998.

Building up the regional role

The second point from the orders that needs underlining with respect to public health concerns measures to allow the regions a greater say in their health affairs. Since the introduction of the April 1996 orders, the "Agences régionales de l'hospitalisation" (ARH) (Regional Hospitalisation Agencies) and "Unions régionales des caisses d'assurance maladie" (URCAM) (Regional Unions of Branches of the National Health Insurance Agency) have been added to the already existing structures, such as the "Directions régionales des Affaires sanitaires et sociales" (DRASS) (Regional Divisions of the Social, Health and Welfare Affairs Directorate), the "Caisses régionales d'assurance maladie" (CRAM) (Regional Branches of the National Health Insurance Agency), the "Unions régionales de médecins libéraux" (URML) (Regional Unions of Physicians in Private Practice), the "Observatoires régionaux de la santé" (ORS) (Regional Health Surveillance Centres), the "Comités régionaux d'éducation pour la santé" (CRES) (Regional Committees for Health Education), etc. This role of co-ordination and stimulation is reinforced by the action of the Regional Health Congresses and their standing committee presided over by the regional "Préfet" (administrator). This trend is also sufficiently compelling for organisations without any "official" regional representation, such as Branches of the "Mutualité sociale agricole" (Agricultural Employees' Health Insurance Agency), to voluntarily set up regional medical and administrative authorities. However, it should be stressed that this general logic corresponds to a process of devolution and not one of decentralisation, indicating a transfer of State jurisdiction to regional advisory bodies.

Health safety measures have been restructured

In response to public demands following the revelation of several instances of malfunction which called into question the quality of the French health system, there has been a considerable reinforcement of health safety measures in several areas in recent years.

The field of drugs and human products for therapeutic use

As far as drugs are concerned, France set up the "Agence du médicament" (National Agency for Drugs and Medication) as a publicly-owned establishment by the law of 4 January 1993. This Agency must ensure that studies and controls relating to the manufacture, trials, therapeutic properties and use of drugs are carried out in a competent scientific and administratively effective manner so that the health and safety of the population are protected.

The same law also transformed the "Agence française du sang" (French Blood Agency), set up as a public interest group in July 1992, into a publicly-owned establishment. This agency was created within the general framework of the reform in blood transfusion resulting from the "contaminated blood" scandal. The aim of the French Blood Agency is to help in defining and applying a policy devoted to blood transfusion, to control and co-ordinate the activities and management of blood transfusion institutions, and to take responsibility for tasks of general interest so as to ensure maximum possible safety as well as satisfy transfusion requirements, and to promote the ethical incorporation of relevant medical, scientific and technological advances into all transfusion procedures.

According to the terms of the law of 18 January 1994, the "Établissement français des greffes" (French Transplantation Institute) was also created as a publicly-owned establishment to replace the "Association France-Transplant" (French Transplant Association).

All of these arrangements have just been modified by the adoption of a government bill concerning health safety that was under discussion in Parliament at the end of 1997 and start of 1998. The law was promulgated on 1 July 1998 and created a "Comité national de la sécurité sanitaire" (National Health Safety Committee"), an "Agence de sécurité sanitaire des produits de santé" (Agency for the Health Safety of Healthcare Products), and an "Agence de sécurité sanitaire des aliments" (Agency for the Health Safety of Foodstuffs) which assume and broaden the tasks of existing agencies, and an "Institut de veille sanitaire" (Health Surveillance Institute) which transforms the National Public Health Network into a publicly-owned establishment.

Protection of workers and the general population against asbestos-related health risks

Two decrees of 7 February 1996 increased the level of protection against asbestos-related health risks. The first decree obliges the owners of premises to search for the presence of flocking, lagging and false ceilings containing asbestos, depending on the building's age. If asbestos is found to be present, the owners must either set up measures for monitoring the situation if the buildings are not too dilapidated, or undertake repair work if they are in a poor state.

The second decree increases worker protection against risks linked to the inhalation of asbestos dust. It differentiates between the various prevention techniques, defines the regulations that apply to de-flocking, tightens the permissible levels of exposure, backs a preventive approach and medical surveillance, and extends the right to compensation.

The right to breathe clean air

The clean air law voted in December 1996 introduced a new right for every French citizen – that of *"breathing air that is not injurious to health"*. Various measures were set out so as to make it possible to exercise this right. In the first place, the measures concern the monitoring of air quality which must be expanded to cover the entire country by the year 2000. More pollutants must be included in the monitoring procedure and the public must be given full details, particularly if pollution thresholds are exceeded.

The law also stipulates that the targets to be achieved in terms of air quality must be defined within the framework of an appropriate regional clean air plan, plans for protection of the atmosphere and plans for urban travel. Travel plans have to be worked out for built-up areas of more than 100,000 inhabitants and must redefine the balance between public and private transport.

Finally, the circulation of traffic can be restricted when pollution levels are high and drivers will be encouraged to use the least polluting vehicles. In 1997, measures to restrict traffic circulation were applied for the first time in France, in Paris and surrounding regions.

Health on a European scale

The limited legal and budgetary framework for health questions

As mentioned recently by the European Commission, the health situations in member countries of the European Union resemble one another in many respects: life expectancy is long, epidemic diseases common in the last century such as smallpox and cholera have disappeared, they also have similar, notable levels of premature mortality (primarily due to lifestyle-related illnesses), new risks of infection have emerged or former risks such as tuberculosis have returned, geographic and social disparities and inequalities still exist and, lastly, they have seen an increase in the number of individuals suffering from diseases and disabilities that are a consequence of old age.

The parallel is even more striking when the challenges faced by member states are considered:
– increase in health expenditure,
– demographic trends (ageing),
– technological advances and their effect on the supply of health care,
– pressures on health systems,
– expectations and concerns of citizens,
– effect of unemployment on health status.

Other additional challenges are the enlargement of the European Union and the spread of problems on a world-wide scale – whose major impact is still too vaguely perceived.

Part one Background to the health situation

Article 129 of the Treaty of Maastricht established a community-wide scope to public health. But it took thirty five years to reach this point and the scope is still limited since it sets out one guideline – *"the Community must assist in ensuring a high level of protection to human health"* – and restricts its targets to prevention and the means employed, practically, to actions of encouragement. Moreover, although an indication is given that *"health requirements are a component of other Community policies"*, the tools for implementing this obligation are lacking.

Actions so far carried out basically concern the following:
– programmes for prevention (cancer, narcotics and substance abuse, AIDS, health promotion) which accompany the best initiatives in the field,
– the formation of a network among public and private public health partners,
– a search for data and indicators which would make it possible to reach an understanding of community-wide determinants of better health and, through them, the impact of other policies,
– preparation of a network for monitoring and controlling transmissible diseases.

Financial resources are limited (250 million francs per annum, *i.e.* approximately 38 million euros, for fifteen member States). However, the principle of subsidiarity only permits Community intervention as a complement to member States – who bear sole responsibility for their health system – and only when its intervention has any actual additional value: this hinders any further achievements in the current situation.

Increasing consideration of the European scale of affairs

The "mad cow" crisis had profound repercussions on European opinion, the governments of member States, scientists, and authorities. Confidence in community organisations had always been somewhat restrained and suffered a further minor setback. So that upon completion of a detailed inquiry, the European Parliament was ready to ask the Court of Justice of the Communities to condemn the Commission in the mad cow affair!

The Commission was so organised that the functions of scientific appraisal and conception and inspection of the implementation of regulations were concentrated under one authority. This made it impossible either to arrive at scientifically sound decisions, or resist political pressures, or check that each member State had applied the prescribed measures. Accordingly, the Commission underwent a reorganisation. The directorate responsible for the protection of consumers and their health (DG XXIV) now has, in addition to a scientific steering committee, eight scientific committees composed of 16 to 18 experts recruited for their competence and under obligation to be independent. At the other end of the decision-making process, operations involved in inspection will be stepped up and coordinated. These measures are designed to check that the control systems of member States are efficient and function in the same manner. The Commission's technical directorates (for industry, agriculture, the domestic market, health, etc.) must conduct their policies with due regard to protecting consumers and their health and give further thought to the exercise of caution. French thinking regarding health safety and the setting up of relevant agencies (health surveillance, healthcare products, foodstuffs) therefore shows great similarity to the course that has been followed in the community.

Reforms should not be restricted to the area of foodstuffs. Both public opinion and public health authorities, who are presently searching for a new framework to include measures that ought to be adopted, are aware that health conditions largely depend on decisions taken in connection with other policies. The latter exert an ever greater influence on the different national regulations as shown by the following few examples which are currently under study:
– prohibition of advertising for smoking, and a common agricultural policy regarding tobacco production,
– asbestos,
– protection against non ionising radiation,
– limits for lead and heavy metals in drinking water,
– limits for atmospheric pollutants;
and, in the realm of health goods:
– safety of drugs derived from components of bovine origin,
– safety of laboratory reagents.

It is therefore important that member States take concerted action in compiling community data bases that will allow the health authorities to defend public health in negotiating these dossiers and to subsequently monitor their impact on public health. French reflections on the appointed tasks of the Health Surveillance Institute have therefore been confirmed and placed in a wider context.

The same sensitivity in opinion and the recent epidemics which have had to be faced (Ebola virus, Hong Kong 'flu) account for the insistence of most member States on the rapid setting up of a European network for controlling transmissible diseases (which will extend to the monitoring of threats to health). The aim is to facilitate as far as possible the co-ordination of replies from health authorities, although the Community has no competence of its own in this area. Yet again, national and community efforts will be mutually supportive.

Health and the Treaty of Amsterdam

Subject to its ratification, the Treaty of Amsterdam will provide a more solid base for the guidelines which have just been mentioned and thereby effectively broaden the area of community action. In fact, the concept of health "improvement" goes beyond the idea of simply preventing illness. Prevention of the "causes of danger" opens up the path to acting on the determinants of health. The idea of prevention will be complete (primary, secondary and tertiary) and the fight against drug addiction could include the "effects" of addiction on health and not just prevention. Measures could be taken in terms of the quality and safety of organs and substances of human origin (including blood). Measures covering veterinary and phytotherapeutic products could be introduced if their prime objective is seen to be the preservation of health, whereas up until now they have been taken within the context of agricultural policy. Lastly, the Treaty states in detail that a high level protection for human health must be ensured *"in defining and implementing all the policies and actions of the Community"*. It will therefore provide a sound basis for reflection on the determinants of health.

Changes are also occurring in the means for appropriate action. In addition to the recommendations and exhortations which already exist, it will be possible to take *"measures laying down high quality and safety standards"* where organs and substances of human origin are concerned. It remains to be seen what form these standards will take since individual member States might adopt measures that are stricter or different.

The Community and healthcare systems

On three occasions, the future Article 152 of the Treaty of Amsterdam underlines national responsibilities and states that community action should "complete" that of member States. Does this arrangement go so far as to restrict or prohibit national healthcare systems from influencing one another? It would seem that the opposite is true.

The recent "Decker" decree of the Court of Justice of the European Communities concerning the compulsory reimbursement of medical expenses for services prescribed in one State and delivered in another will certainly have repercussions on the autonomy of health systems, both in terms of financial management and the quality of services that each offers. However, regardless of this aspect, there is a tendency towards rapprochement. The Commission proposes to place the following on the list of exchanges to be encouraged between member States: data on health systems, their reform, and the most successful experiments carried out to restrain costs, foster competition, and improve the quality and efficacy of services.

An informal meeting of Ministers for Health was organised in July 1998 by the Austrian presidency concerning quality assurance in public health, particularly in hospitals. Other presidencies intend to get the ministers to discuss specific facets of their health system (mental health, online health services, etc.).

Thus, member States are going beyond the mere co-ordination of their policies of prevention enjoined by Article 129 of the Treaty of Maastricht and are gradually fitting their actions involving public health and health system reform into an increasingly convergent framework. It is therefore advisable to ask whether the various parties involved in public health policy in France have come to all the right conclusions regarding organisation and means of implementation.

CHAPTER TWO

Public opinions and perceptions

An understanding of the public's perception of its health status, the common meanings of "good health", and public expectations in terms of prevention and the general conduct of health policies are all factors which are part and parcel of baseline data included in reflections concerning the country's health situation. A large number of surveys on health also include questions about perceived health. In order to tackle this topic in greater detail during preparation of the present report, the High Committee on Public Health had the "Centre de recherche pour l'étude et l'observation des conditions de vie" (CREDOC: Centre for Research and Surveillance of Standards of Living)[1] carry out a specific inquiry into the subject, as it had previously done for the report published in 1994.

The public's perception of its health status is highly satisfactory on the whole and has not altered appreciably since 1992.

Overall persistently high public satisfaction with health

In late 1997, 89% of those questioned replied that their state of health was satisfactory or very satisfactory in comparison with that of others of the same age. Basically, this opinion varied according to the age of the person questioned: 95% of those in the 20-34 years age bracket and 76% of those over 70 were globally satisfied. The effect of age is especially obvious in figure 1.

It can particularly be seen that the reply "very satisfactory" was given by one third of those interviewed in the 20 to 34 years age group and only one eighth of those aged over 65. Men claimed to be in a slightly better state of health than women.

---

1. Le Quéau P., Olm C., "*La perception de la santé en France*" (Perception of health in France), a study carried out at the request of the High Committee on Public Health, CREDOC, collection of reports, No. 85, January 1998, 134 p.
The study was conducted in October 1997 and consisted of a telephone interview of a sample of 2,017 persons aged over 20, obtained by the method of quotas that took into consideration age, sex, size of the district of residence, region of residence and socioprofessional category. The previous survey had been carried out under similar conditions in 1992.

Part one Background to the health situation

Figure 1 **Perception of health status as a function of age**

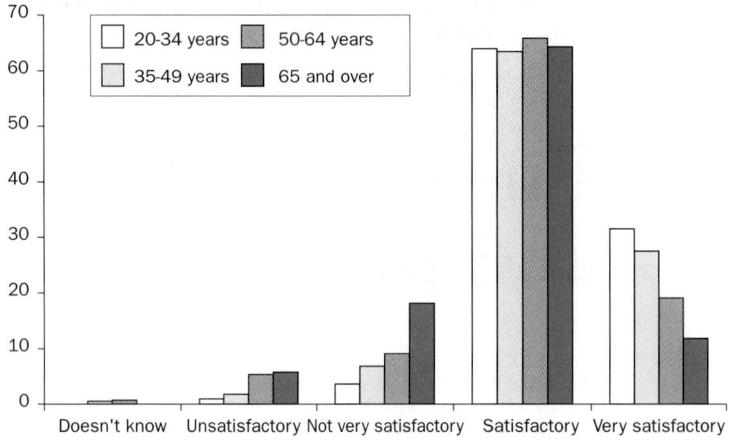

- 20-34 years
- 35-49 years
- 50-64 years
- 65 and over

Categories (x-axis): Doesn't know, Unsatisfactory, Not very satisfactory, Satisfactory, Very satisfactory

Source: HCSP/Credoc, 1997.

Although the persons questioned declared that their state of health was satisfactory on the whole, the statement has to be qualified in terms of the interviewee's social situation. Compared with those in employment, half as many of the unemployed declared themselves very satisfied with their health status (16% *versus* 29%), and three times as many stated that they were dissatisfied (17% *versus* 6%). It is significant that, in spite of the age difference, their replies matched those among the retired. Among those in the labour force and in actual employment, 33% of management and those in liberal professions considered themselves very satisfied with their state of health compared with 24% of employees and manual workers. This correlation with social situation is clearly evident in terms of income. For example, one quarter of those interviewed over 50 years of age living in a household with an income of over 15,000 francs regarded their health status as very satisfactory compared with only 7% of those in the same age bracket and living in a household with a combined income of not more than 4,000 francs.

The way in which the enquiry was conducted (by telephone) excluded a marginalised portion of the population and the elderly living in institutions. These global data are therefore slightly overestimated and doubtless mask some situations which, although limited in number, are particularly difficult. Moreover, since an opinion survey is involved, the mode of questioning is very important *(see box)* and the replies reflect an entire set of perceptions specific to the particular group of respondents involved.

Public opinions and perceptions

THE IMPORTANCE OF HOW QUESTIONS ARE FORMULATED

In France, public surveys concerning health generally introduce one question relating to the respondent's perceived health. This makes it possible to compare the replies given according to the manner in which the question is posed.

Most surveys ask respondents to compare themselves with other persons of the same age. This enhances the normative nature of the question and tends to increase the rate of declared satisfaction. However, even if this explicit reference is lacking during questioning, there is obviously an implicit reference to age, as shown by the high level of satisfaction expressed by those in older age brackets. In one ongoing CREDOC survey carried out in connection with the "loi Evin" evaluation, there has been only a 3% difference in the "very satisfactory" replies given by two sub-samples, one of which made reference to persons of the same age while the other omitted the age reference.

Thus, when people were asked about the limitations they perceive in daily life, one third stated that they were very satisfied or satisfied with their state of health, even though they were unable to eat everything they wanted, and above all one person in five expressed the same degree of satisfaction concerning his/her state of health in spite of stated limitations in terms of moving about outside or in the home. It is obvious that these limitations become apparent as people advance in years.

"Moderate" replies particularly illustrate the importance of the phrasing of the questionnaire. A comparison of the results from French surveys, some of which included this item while others did not, shows that the "moderate" reply is divided between one third "not very satisfactory" and two thirds "satisfactory", *i.e.* the two items which bracket "moderate". In the Health Barometer of the "Comité français d'éducation pour la santé" (CFES) (French Health Education Committee), the "satisfactory" item was replaced by "fairly satisfactory". Comparison of the results from the CFES and CREDOC surveys showed that simply adding "fairly" led to a 5% increase in the replies for this item at the expense of the item "very satisfactory".

Changes over the last decade regarded as very positive, especially by the elderly

Two thirds of those interviewed felt that the health status of the French had improved over the last ten years. The percentage of positive replies showed a slight increase relative to the 1992 survey. This opinion was notably affected by the subject's own state of health: 32% of those dissatisfied with their own health status considered that the collective health status had deteriorated compared with 22% of respondents as a whole. Men were more positive in their assessment of changes undergone (66% of men felt there had been an improvement compared with 61% of women, 19% of men considered that a deterioration had occurred compared with 24% of women). A negative view of the past was adopted far more frequently by the youngest respondents and, more generally, by those under fifty years old. In contrast, those who were older, and especially retired people, took a much more positive view of the past decade, only 15% believing that the situation had got worse compared with 70% who felt it had improved. It may be that a considerable fringe of those who are young or of average age are particularly sensitive to recent health crises – including AIDS – and programmes to promote awareness of risks, unlike those who are older and find it easier to put the recent past into perspective. For some, a realisation that the social situation among the young has taken a downturn might also play a role.

Being unemployed actually encourages a much more negative view of past changes (39% *versus* 23% for those in employment) even among those who have a positive perception of their own condition.

A less optimistic view of future changes in the health status of the population

The picture of the future is far less optimistic than the backward glance over the past decade: although one person in two thinks that the state of public health will improve over the next decade, 30% assume the opposite. Obviously, this view is also affected by each individual's perception of his own health status: thus, 39% of those dissatisfied with their personal state of health foresee a future deterioration in the collective health status compared with 28% of all those interviewed. However, a certain cautiousness could be discerned in the replies; 20% of those interviewed felt that the collective health status would remain identical in the coming decade and 36% that it would show a slight improvement. Only one person in eight optimistically declared "the state of health of French people will improve a great deal", whereas three out of ten thought that this had been the case in the last ten years. Similarly, men were slightly more confident than women; on the other hand, there was no apparent age-based difference. The difference in past/future perception is therefore particularly marked among the elderly. This may be the effect of each individual's perception of the changes in his own health on that of future health progression in the population as a whole.

The markedly less optimistic view of the future health status of the French may be connected with the fact that social factors are increasingly taken into account as determinants of health status, as analysed below. It may also be related to the public's far more acute awareness of environment-related risks. Hence, according to the annual "barometric survey" of risks and safety carried out by the IPSN (Institut de protection et de sûreté nucléaire = Institute for Nuclear Safety and Protection), between May 1996 and November 1997, the percentage of individuals who answered "yes" to the question "do you or your loved ones feel personally threatened by atmospheric pollution" rose from 58% to 66%, "... by water pollution" from 56% to 69%, "... by the hole in the ozone layer" from 47% to 62%. More generally, 81% considered that the population was increasingly exposed to multiple risks. This rapid change in the perception of environmental risks might be one factor that accounts for a less sanguine view of the collective future than of past changes.

An altered perception of what constitutes "good health" since 1992, particularly among management

When asked what it means to them, people practically always associate good health with a feeling of well-being and autonomy (table 1).

Equating good health with a long life span already raises additional questions and only one person in two completely agrees with this assertion. It may be noted that workers are more "strongly" in agreement (65% compared with 50% among the rest of the population), which seems to indicate that their perception reflects a disadvantage in terms of life expectancy. In 1997, the negative notions of "not being ill" and "not suffering" which received the same approval rating as "living better" in 1992, were rated more highly – as high or almost as high as the positive items "well-being" and "autonomy". This is one of the main differences noted in the results of the two surveys. It was accompanied by greater uniformity in the replies of the general population since the change particularly concerned management personnel who, in 1992, devoted greater importance to positive than negative notions of good health, negative notions apparently being more widespread among the less affluent.

This change was confirmed by the survey already mentioned and conducted by CREDOC in 1998 as part of the assessment of the "loi Evin" (Evin law which restricted the conditions for advertising alcohol). Respondents were asked to arrange various items with a positive connotation (being fit, enjoying life) and negative connotation (not being ill, not suffering) in order of priority.

"Being fit" was rated first by 31% of those interviewed and "not being ill" by 27%. The first and second choice items were recorded respectively as "being fit, and enjoying life" for 10% of respondents, while 9% gave "not being ill, and being fit" as their respective first and second choices.

It is hard to do more than make assumptions in interpreting the results from opinion polls. Several broad explanatory factors might be advanced in discussing the change that has taken place, including the more general shifts in public opinion as a result of socio-economic movements in society during the period 1992-1997. By analogy, it might be supposed that the fear of

Part one Background to the health situation

Table 1 **Replies given in 1992 and 1997 to the question: "Do you associate good health with…"**
(as a percentage)

	1992	1997
Enjoying life		
Strongly	88	85
A little	11	13
Not at all	1	1
Doing what one likes		
Strongly	80	83
A little	18	15
Not at all	1	3
Not being ill		
Strongly	63	82
A little	27	15
Not at all	10	3
Not suffering		
Strongly	57	74
A little	32	19
Not at all	11	7
Not having to see a doctor		
Strongly	40	45
A little	35	36
Not at all	26	19
Having a long life		
Strongly	60	53
A little	28	34
Not at all	8	13

Source: HCSP/Credoc, 1997.

illness corresponds to the fear of unemployment, another "negative" concept which has spread (particularly among management) to the detriment of "positive" work-associated values.

Other explanations could be suggested without going outside the sphere of health. Public opinion has without doubt acquired a certain consciousness as a result of repeated health crises, bad news (proven or otherwise) concerning fresh risks or the resurgence of risks that were thought to have been brought under control, unlike the linear effects of never-ending announcements of medical and scientific progress. Under the stimulus of an explosive development in health-devoted media, it is not surprising that an absence of illness is once again being seen as an essential factor in "good health".

Increased perception of social factors as determinants of health status

In 1997 as in 1992, nutrition and pollution were regarded as preponderant determinants of health status. The only slight difference concerns the degree of support among those who fully agreed or were fairly much in agreement, although practically no disagreement was expressed (1 to 2%). Among the youngest age brackets and among men, 15 to 20% of respondents avoided giving a completely cut-and-dried opinion.

The same characteristics were found in judgements concerning alcohol consumption and smoking. The proposal to further curb alcohol consumption and smoking received massive backing (81% of those surveyed said they fully agreed, 14% were fairly much in agreement, and only 5% were against). Again, it was among the young, especially young males, that hesitation or refusal were encountered, while the degree of support showed a regular increase with age. Thus, the current almost general consensus is that smoking and alcohol are harmful: this was confirmed by the CFES ("Comité français d'éducation pour la santé", French Health Education Committee) health barometer which found that 90% of the French consider that smokers are as dependent on tobacco as on a drug, and the majority of smokers (86%) concur in this opinion.

The significance of this consensus must therefore be tempered by the respondents' highly variable perception of the harmfulness of smoking and alcohol. In fact, the survey carried out by CREDOC within the scope of the previously mentioned evaluation of the Evin law reported that replies put the average number of cigarettes smoked daily and considered as dangerous to health at eight – which means that an appreciable proportion of those interviewed quoted a much higher figure. This indicates the difficulty that smokers and drinkers experience in switching from an abstract response to a general question to the reduction or cessation of their own consumption, and also the need to improve the population's understanding of the actual deleterious effects of these products.

Social and living conditions are the other major set of factors regarded as affecting an individual's state of health. Conditions concerning housing, working, training, transport safety and family isolation are very largely perceived as determinants of health, though certainly to a lesser extent than nutrition and the environment. These facts had already been noted in the 1992 survey (table 2).

The most remarkable change since 1992 concerns uncertainty (unemployment, lack of money). Admittedly, fewer than 10% of those interviewed in the 1992 survey disagreed with the idea that these factors played a role in influencing health status, but 30% expressed limited agreement ("fairly much in agreement"). A shift in opinion was evident in 1997 and 73% of respondents replied that they fully agreed that unemployment affected health and 67% that a lack of money also played a role. In addition, the replies from various social groups were more homogeneous, the greatest change being noted among management and those with the highest incomes (+ 15%).

Table 2 **Replies given in 1992 and 1997 to the question: "Do you think the following problems affect health?"**

	1992	1997
Being unemployed		
Fully agree	61	73
Fairly in agreement	29	21
Not having enough money		
Fully agree	59	67
Fairly in agreement	31	26
Isolation from children		
Fully agree	45	54
Fairly in agreement	37	33
Feeling of insecurity		
Fully agree	45	46
Fairly in agreement	37	34
Lack of training		
Fully agree	36	34
Fairly in agreement	32	34
Distance between home and work		
Fully agree	36	44
Fairly in agreement	39	37
Living alone all the time		
Fully agree	33	34
Fairly in agreement	36	33

Source: HCSP/Credoc, 1997.

As in 1992, 67% of people felt that increasing the number of doctors would not bring about any improvement in health status. This percentage was lower among the most modest social groups and respondents professing a poor state of health and therefore had a greater need for healthcare, but remained well above 50% in all cases.

Opinions concerning prevention were consistent with the above findings. Three quarters of respondents agreed that the attention devoted to nutrition and improving the environment contributed to prevention and the remaining quarter was fairly much in agreement; as for an improvement in working conditions, one half and a little under 40% respectively agreed and fairly much agreed that this contributed to prevention. In the strictly medical domain, keeping up-to-date with vaccinations was regarded as preventive by 75% (fully agree) and 19% (fairly much in agreement) of individuals; the respective proportions were 53% and 33% in terms of regular follow-up by a doctor. Opinions on prevention have seen considerable changes where screening education programmes are concerned. Between 1992 and 1997, those who fully agreed that such programmes contribute to prevention jumped from 56 to 75% and those who disagreed dropped from 10 to 4%.

In 1997, external factors (social and environmental) were perceived to play a greater role in the health status of the population than in 1992. However, this does not shatter the widely held view that maintaining the health status of the population is the personal responsibility of each individual – an opinion that received the full agreement of 69% of those questioned (77% in 1992), while those who replied that they were fairly much in agreement rose from 17% in 1992 to 27% in 1997.

Any priority must be given to the destitute

The public is practically equally divided over the question of whether the State should grant priority to certain groups among the population as part of its health policy. Opinions on this point have remained consistently steady since 1992, the only difference appearing in women over 35 who, unlike men, mostly agreed that the State should grant priority.

The most destitute were overwhelmingly singled out as the population group which should be accorded *priority*, whereas "the elderly" were not often selected (table 3). Young people between the ages of 20 and 34 were the most sympathetic to the plight of "destitute individuals".

It is impossible to measure any change in opinion on this point relative to 1992 since "the most destitute" was not listed as an optional group among the replies in the 1992 survey. The simple fact that this item was inserted since the last survey was carried out indicates that the concerns of society have undergone a transformation.

Table 3 **Priority to be given by the State to certain population groups in its health policy, answers according to age**
(as a percentage)

	20-34 years	35-49 years	50-64 years	65 and over	Total
Newborn	8	4	4	6	5
Young people (18 to 25)	4	8	6	9	6
Elderly	2	2	3	5	3
Handicapped	4	4	6	8	5
Most destitute	28	26	22	19	25
None of the above	2	1	1	2	2
No priority to be given	52	55	58	51	54

Source: HCSP/Credoc, 1997.

Part one Background to the health situation

Poor perception of the region as the site of health policy implementation

As far as the population is concerned, health questions are unimportant on a regional scale and no different from all other political questions in this respect. Only 10% of those questioned felt that health policy should primarily be implemented at the regional level. Two thirds of respondents mentioned that the national and European levels were important (36% and 29% respectively) and, in keeping with the usual political sociology, the district council (16%) came ahead of the region (10%) and department (8%).

The distribution of opinions was unaffected by either sex or age, although the European level was mentioned slightly more frequently by the young. Among the unemployed, the choice of the national level (44%) and the nearest site, the district council (19%), was above average. Only management gave slightly greater importance to the region (21%).

There was practically no variation in the distribution of replies between 1992 and 1997 and this steadiness was altogether conspicuous since, during this interval and as far as health was concerned, the regional level had been given strong political backing by the publication of the 1996 edicts, the holding of regional health congresses, and the setting up of Regional Agencies for Hospitalisation.

In conclusion, greater receptiveness to public health topics

In 1997, an improvement in personal health status and that of the population at large was regarded primarily as a question of adopting a healthy lifestyle – there was plenty of scope for reducing individual risk factors, but each person's social and physical environment also exerted an effect. This change appears to be underpinned by growing anxiety over a perceived rise in socio-economic problems and environmental risks. The public seems to have a better appreciation of the importance of screening and health education programmes.

PART TWO

Changes
in health status

CHAPTER THREE

Indicators of health status

This chapter introduces a clear separation between so-called **general** indicators of the population's state of health and specific indicators corresponding to particular areas of health or particular groups amongst the population. In fact, this distinction is quite evident in the 1994 report and is tacitly adopted in most reports on health status drawn up abroad.

General indicators are diagnostic tools for health problems at the national, regional or local levels. In fact, an enduring standstill in life expectancy, life expectancy with unimpaired health lower than that in a neighbouring region, an increasing number of potential years of life wasted because of road accidents, etc. are all possible examples of signals for detecting health problems in a population. Only the availability of information and the size of the populations concerned might prove to be factors limiting the use of such indicators, many of which – not by chance – rely on demographic data and national statistics concerning the causes of death. However, the development of more refined, and hence more useful, indicators may involve additional data which are not routinely compiled. This is why changes in life expectancy with unimpaired health in France during the last period could not be studied in the present report. Data concerning the prevalence of disability available on a representative statistical data base were actually derived from the last decennial INSEE survey on health carried out in 1991. General indicators relating to morbidity stated by the population or morbidity treated by the healthcare system are also available, even if they are difficult to interpret since they depend in large measure on the care proposed.

There are potentially very large numbers of **specific indicators** of health status, whether they concern measurements of physical or mental well-being, good social adjustment, the prevalence or incidence of symptoms or illnesses, the frequency of death from specific causes, etc. It can be seen that to a large extent the choice of indicators is closely linked with the definition of top priority health areas. The High Committee on Public Health decided to go over the top priority health problems described in the second part of the 1994 report and analyse the changes in the corresponding indicators during the last few years, comparing them with targets that were set at the time for the year 2000 (or sometimes 2010).

The following three areas have not been considered in this chapter since recent specific indicators were unobtainable when the present work was being drafted: iatrogenic illness and nosocomial infections[1], child abuse, and pain. It should be noted that the 1994 report insisted on the pressing need to dispose of reliable quantitative information for each of these areas: however, this call was apparently unheard. This does not mean that public authorities have failed to take any initiative to trigger progress in the area concerned during this period – this is particularly true in the case of the fight against pain which is being tackled in a three-year pain relief plan (1998-2000).

General indicators

Changes in mortality and life expectancy

Major gains in life expectancy have been made since the 1980s but there is a tendency to tail off

The life expectancy of the French population continues to make headway. In 1996, it was 74 years for men and 82 years for women (table 1). Between 1991 and 1996, a mean annual increase of 2.5 months per year was noted for men and 2 months for women. This points out not only the large gap still dividing the sexes but also its slight tendency to shrink (7.9 years in 1996 and 8.2 years in 1991). The increase in life expectancy noted at the beginning of the 1990s is less than that observed during the decade of the 80s (gain of 3 months per year for both sexes). In particular, a slowdown in increasing life expectancy has been noted after the age of 60.

---

1. It should be recalled that this topic was selected as one of 10 priorities by the "Conférence nationale de santé" (CNS) (National Health Congress) 1996 and was discussed at the CNS 1998. A contribution from the HCSP *"Contribution aux réflexions sur la lutte contre l'iatrogénie"* (Contribution to reflections on the fight against iatrogenesis) was also discussed at the CNS and in Parliament.

Table 1 **Life expectancy in France at birth and at 60 years (1996, 1991 and 1981) according to sex**

	Men	Women
Life expectancy at birth		
1996	74.0	81.9
1991	72.9	81.1
1981	70.4	78.5
Annual gain 1981-1991	0.25	0.26
Annual gain 1991-1996	0.22	0.16
Life expectancy at 60 years		
1996	19.7	25.0
1991	19.2	24.4
1981	17.3	22.3
Annual gain 1981-1991	0.19	0.21
Annual gain 1991-1996	0.10	0.12

Source: Insee.

Increased life expectancy with unimpaired health which has to be confirmed over a recent period

The appreciable increase in life expectancy since the 1980s has raised an important question concerning changes in the overall health status of the population. Are these additional years of life spent in good health or accompanied by excessive disabilities? This interrogation led to the drawing up of a specific indicator, "life expectancy with unimpaired health" (LEUH). As its name implies, this indicator covers both life expectancy and the prevalence of disabilities in a given population.

Although life expectancy increased by 2.5 years between 1981 and 1991, life expectancy with unimpaired health showed a greater rise (3.0 years for men and 2.6 years for women)[2] and there was an increase in the proportion of life span with unimpaired health. Contrary to frequently expressed fears concerning growing disability, expanding life expectancy was accompanied by "shrinking morbidity". This reduction in disability among the elderly cannot be attributed to less prevalent incapacitating chronic illnesses since the latter have been shown to be undergoing a parallel increase. On the other hand, the most frequent chronic illnesses (cardiovascular, bone and joint diseases, etc.) are tending to become less disabling. However, these results must be interpreted with caution since the measurement of change is based on the patient's own appreciation of his disabilities.

Life expectancy with unimpaired health is a highly informative indicator in complementing life expectancy data. However, it can only be calculated when regular data concerning disability among the population are available, and this is not presently the case (latest data available are from the 1990 INSEE survey). Hence, gains in

---

2. Robine J.M., Mormiche P., *"L'espérance de vie sans incapacité augmente"* (The length of life expectancy with unimpaired health is increasing), INSEE Première, 1993, 281.

Part two   Changes in health status

life expectancy with unimpaired health will have to be confirmed over a more recent period.

The risk of death persistently declining for all age brackets but less markedly among the elderly

In 1996, a total of 535,506 deaths were recorded in metropolitan France. 52% of those who died were men, 21% were under 65 (113,786 deaths) and 2% under 25 (10,356 deaths). In 1991, the corresponding death total was 524,700, including 124,222 under 65-year-olds (24%).

The rise in the number of deaths between 1991 and 1996 was the result of ageing in the structure of the French population. In actual fact, when the death total is expressed relative to the size of the population (mortality rate), a reduction in the risk of death can be seen between 1991 and 1996. The total of 535,506 deaths observed in 1996 corresponds to a mortality rate of 880 per 100,000 inhabitants. This mortality rate, standardised for age, dropped by 6% between 1991 and 1996. The decrease was similar for both sexes and applied to all age brackets, although it varied in amplitude and trend (table 2 and figure 1).

Table 2 **Mortality rate in France in 1996 and variation in mortality rate between 1991 and 1996[a], according to sex and age**
(comparative mortality rate per 100,000 standardised by age, France, both sexes, 1990)

	Men	Women	Total
Total			
1996 rate	1,200.7	655.9	880.1
1991-1996 rate variation	– 5%	– 6%	– 6%
Under 65 years			
1996 rate	328.9	136.8	231.5
1991-1996 rate variation	– 11%	– 8%	– 10%
Under 25 years			
1996 rate	72.4	38.7	55.8
1991-1996 rate variation	– 26%	– 26%	– 26%
25-44 years			
1996 rate	211.8	88.2	149.9
1991-1996 rate variation	– 10%	– 2%	– 8%
45-64 years			
1996 years	919.6	368.3	638.1
1991-1996 rate variation	– 9%	– 6%	– 8%
65-74 years			
1996 rate	2,713.5	1,121.5	1,830.0
1991-1996 rate variation	– 3%	– 4%	– 3%
75 years and over			
1996 rate	10,002.6	6,362.8	7,617.2
1991-1996 rate variation	– 3%	– 6%	– 4%

a. 1991-1996 variation = (1996 rate – 1991 rate)/1991 rate x 100.
Source: Inserm SC8.

Indicators of health status

Figure 1 **Variation in mortality rate as a function of sex and age, 1980-1996**
(comparative mortality rates standardised per 100 000 by age, both sexes, 1990, smoothed curves, provisional 1996 data)

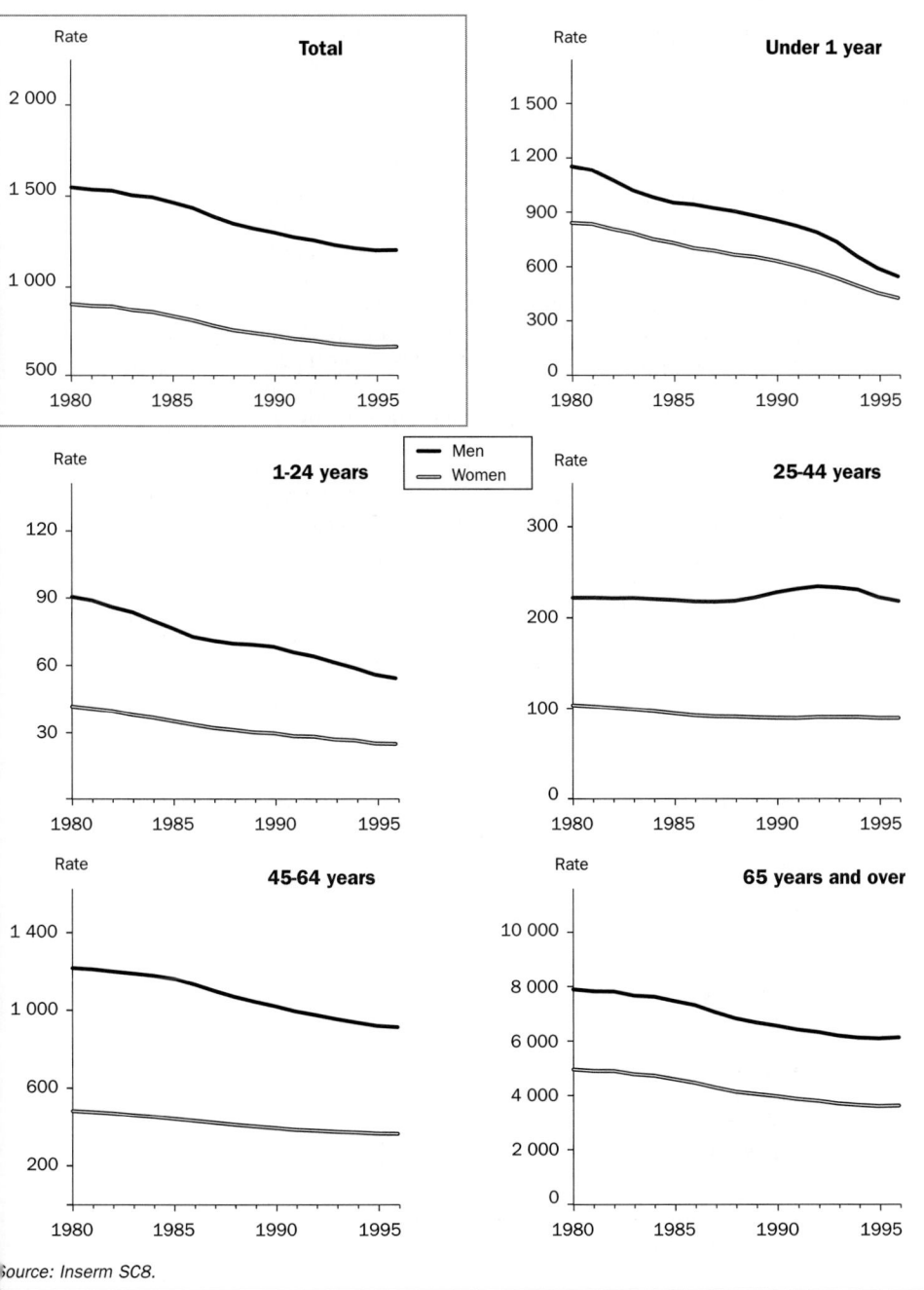

Source: Inserm SC8.

The most marked drops were noted in those under 25 of either sex (– 26%) and, to a lesser extent, in men between 25 and 64 (– 10%). There was little decrease among adult women and men over 65. In the most recent years (1995-1996), the mortality rate has shown a tendency to mark time and even increase slightly in those over 65 (these years were marked by major influenza epidemics).

However, the fall in the mortality rate noted during the period 1991-1996 was smaller than that observed in the previous period (1985-1990). This trend was basically due to a smaller decline in the risk of death among the elderly, whereas premature mortality continued to rise at the same pace.

Cancer is increasing but cardiovascular diseases remain the prime cause of death

The main causes of death are cardiovascular disease (32% of total mortality in 1996), followed by cancer (28%), violent death (9%) and respiratory disease (8%). These proportions vary appreciably, according to sex (table 3). In men, cancer is in the lead (32% *versus* 29% for cardiovascular disease), whereas cardiovascular disease is still widely predominant in women (36% *versus* 23% for cancer). Violent death (suicides, accidents, etc.) accounts for 10% of mortality among men compared with 7% among women.

Table 3 **Number of subjects and percentage of principal diseases involved in mortality, according to sex**
(total number of deaths, 1996 and 1991)

	Men 1996		Women 1996		Total 1996		Total 1991	
	n	%	n	%	n	%	n	%
Cardiovascular disease	79,595	29	93,592	36	173,187	32	175,681	34
Cancer	89,194	32	58,527	23	147,721	28	143,267	27
Violent death	26,279	10	17,402	7	43,681	9	47,206	8
Respiratory disease	22,131	8	20,391	8	42,522	8	36,015	7
Gastrointestinal disease	13,924	5	12,509	5	26,433	5	26,646	5
Other diseases	45,522	16	56,425	21	101,947	18	95,897	19
Total	276,645	100	258,846	100	535,491	100	524,712	100

Source: Inserm SC8.

When "premature" mortality is analysed, the proportion of the various groups of diseases is very different (table 4). In those under 65, deaths are due to: cancer 37%, violence 19%, and cardiovascular disease 15%. In those under 45, 4 out of 10 men and 3 out of 10 women die a violent death (figure 2). Between the ages of 45 and 64, one death in two is due to cancer.

The indicator "potential years of life lost" (PYLL) is an additional gauge of premature mortality which takes into account the degree

Table 4 **Number of subjects and percentage of principal diseases involved in mortality, according to sex**
(premature deaths, before 65 years, 1996 and 1991)

	Men 1996		Women 1996		Total 1996		Total 1991	
	n	%	n	%	n	%	n	%
Cancer	28,180	35	14,329	42	42,509	37	44 623	36
Violent death	16,387	21	5,677	17	22,064	19	25,013	20
Cardiovascular disease	12,549	16	3,995	12	16,544	15	18,966	15
Digestive disease	5,157	7	2,288	7	7,445	7	7,958	6
Respiratory disease	2,508	3	1,025	3	3,533	3	3,614	3
Other diseases	15,006	18	6,685	19	21,691	19	24,048	20
Total	79,787	100	33,999	100	113,786	100	124,222	100

Source: Inserm SC8.

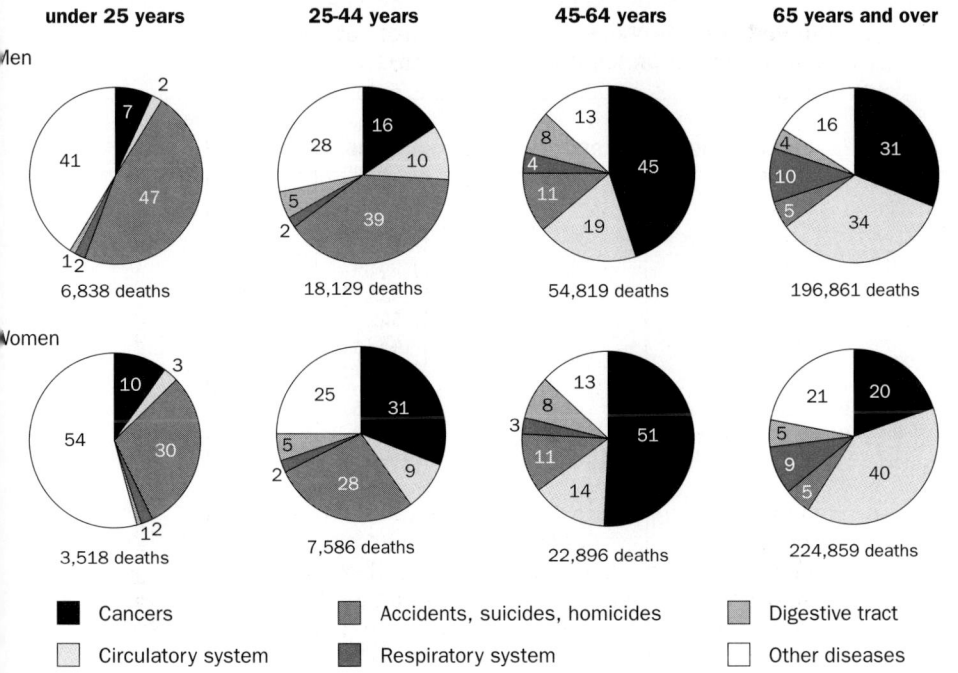

Figure 2 **Percentage of principal diseases responsible for mortality as a function of sex and age group in 1996**

Source: Inserm SC8.

Part two Changes in health status

of prematurity in "premature" deaths. It is defined as the number of potential years of life lost when a subject dies "prematurely", *i.e.* before the age of 65 (for example, someone who dies at age 52 years has lost thirteen potential years of life). In 1996, violent death accounted for one third of the PYLL, cancer for one quarter and cardiovascular disease one tenth (table 5). The relative influence of these major pathological groups varies with sex, 36% of PYLL being due to violent death and 25% to cancer among men, and 34% to cancer and 27% to violent death among women. More detailed analysis reveals the order of importance of death causing the loss of potential years of life; for men, road accidents and suicide, followed by lung cancer, infarction, AIDS and alcoholism; for women, road accidents, suicide and breast cancer.

The distribution of the main causes of death has remained stable since 1991. However, a slight increase in the relative importance of cancer and a parallel decrease in that of violent death has been observed. The same trends have been noted for the components of PYLL (a decrease in the relative importance of road accidents has also been noted since 1991 in PYLL).

Table 5 **Potential years of life lost (from 1 to 64 years) according to the cause of death and sex**
(percentage of principal diseases, 1991 and 1996)

	Total		Men		Women	
	1991	1996	1991	1996	1991	1996
Cancer	25	27	23	25	32	34
including						
Lung cancer	4	5	5	6	2	3
Cancer of the UADT[a]	4	3	5	4	1	1
Breast cancer	3	3			9	9
Uterine cancer	1	1			2	2
Intestinal cancer	1	2	1	1	2	2
Cardiovascular disease	11	11	11	11	9	9
including						
Ischaemic heart disease	4	4	4	5	2	2
Cerebrovascular disease	3	3	2	2	3	3
Violent death	35	33	38	36	29	27
including						
Road accidents	14	11	15	12	11	9
Suicide	10	11	11	12	8	9
Cirrhosis, alcoholic psychosis	5	5	5	5	5	5
Diseases of the respiratory system	2	2	2	2	3	3
AIDS	5	5	6	5	3	4
Other causes	17	17	15	16	19	18
Total	**100**	**100**	**100**	**100**	**100**	**100**

a. Cancer of the upper airways and digestive tract (including oesophagus).
Source: Inserm SC8.

Indicators of health status

Reduction in the risk of death from most diseases other than cancers related to smoking and alcoholism in women

During the period 1991-1996, the risk of death linked to most diseases continued to decline (table 6). The most marked fall was noted in violent deaths, with a particularly important drop in road accident fatalities (more marked among men). In contrast, the decrease in the suicide rate was moderate and slowed down at the start of the 1990s. The mortality rates due to various cardiovascular diseases also showed a distinct fall (more pronounced drop in cerebral vascular accidents than infarctions). The mortality rates directly linked to alcoholism continued to fall sharply but not as sharply as before.

Table 6 **Variation in mortality rate as a function of the principal diseases between 1991 and 1996 and sex**
(comparative mortality rate per 100,000 standardised by age[a], 1990)

	Total mortality		"Premature" mortality (before 65 years)	
	Men	Women	Men	Women
Cardiovascular disease	– 8%	– 12%	– 14%	– 16%
Cancer	– 4%	– 2%	– 8%	– 3%
Violent death	– 11%	– 14%	– 14%	– 11%
Respiratory disease	+ 5%	+ 9%	– 3%	– 3%
Cirrhosis, alcoholic psy.	– 10%	– 10%	– 12%	– 11%
AIDS	– 12%	+ 36%	– 12%	+ 44%
Total	– 5%	– 6%	– 11%	– 8%

a. 1991-1996 variation = (1996 rate – 1991 rate)/1991 rate x 100.
Source: Inserm SC8.

The cancer-related mortality rates tended to stand still (although certain locations continued to show a strong decline, such cancers of the stomach and uterus). The most noteworthy phenomenon was a considerable progression in tobacco- and alcohol-related cancers in women: + 20% for lung cancer and an increase in cancers of the upper airways and digestive tract (UADT) among elderly women. The situation with respect to these diseases was very different among men: lung cancer stopped increasing and cancers of the UADT continued to decline sharply.

Since 1991, an augmentation has been noted in the mortality rates due to respiratory diseases, essentially among the elderly (influenza epidemics in 1995 and 1996). AIDS-related mortality continued to climb among women after 1991 but decreased among men. However, starting from 1996, a reduction in the mortality rate due to AIDS has been observed for both sexes. In contrast, an increase has recently been noted in some specific diseases such as different types of hepatitis and melanoma.

Part two — Changes in health status

Persistent, particularly high excess mortality among men

The general mortality rate (standardised for age) is almost twice as high among men as it is among women (table 7). The magnitude of this difference remains a specifically French feature (it is the highest, relative to other European countries). The most marked difference between the sexes occurs between the ages of 25 and 74 years (risk of death multiplied by a factor of 2.5), whereas after 74 years, excess mortality among males is only 1.5. The difference between the sexes has remained stable since 1991 with a slight tendency to rise among those over 65 and to fall among those aged between 25 and 64.

Table 7 **Excess mortality among men according to age, in 1996 and 1991**
(ratio of male/female rates standardised for age)

	1996	1991
Total	1.83	1.81
under 25 years	1.87	1.86
25-44 years	2.40	2.64
45-64 years	2.50	2.58
65-74 years	2.42	2.39
75 years and over	1.57	1.53

Source: Inserm SC8.

The maximum differences in the risk of death between men and women are found in terms of cancers of the upper airways and digestive tract and lung cancers (table 8). Excess mortality among men is still staggering for these diseases (risk of death among males multiplied respectively by 9 and 7 and, for deaths before the age of 65, by 11 and 7). These are followed by (risks multiplied by more than 2 among men): AIDS, suicide, alcoholism, road accidents, carcinomas of the stomach, infarctions and respiratory diseases.

While the overall level of excess mortality among men may have varied very little since 1991, there is still a trend towards a smaller difference between the sexes in terms of some diseases (cancers of the upper airways and digestive tract, lung cancer and AIDS).

Particularly high "avoidable" mortality related to risk behaviour among men

As in the earlier report, two types of indicator have been differentiated for "premature" mortality (under the age of 65), (table 9):
– "avoidable" deaths linked to individual risk behaviours; causes of death whose incidence could essentially be decreased by acting on individual behaviours (risks related to smoking, alcohol consumption, dangerous driving, etc.); this selection includes lung cancers, cancers of the upper airways and digestive tract, alcoholism, road accidents, suicides and AIDS;

Table 8 **Excess mortality among men as a function of the principal diseases**
(ratio of male/female mortality rates standardised for age, France, 1996 and 1991)

	Total mortality		"Premature" mortality (before 65 years)	
	1996	1991	1996	1991
All causes	1.8	1.8	2.4	2.5
Cancer	2.2	2.3	2.0	2.2
including				
Cancer of the UADT[a]	8.7	10.7	11.3	13.3
Lung cancer	7.2	8.6	6.9	9.3
Intestinal cancer	1.7	1.7	1.6	1.6
Stomach carcinoma	2.5	2.4	3.0	3.1
Cardiovascular disease	1.6	1.6	3.3	3.2
including				
Infarction	2.2	2.1	6.2	5.7
Stroke	1.4	1.3	1.9	2.0
Violent death	2.2	2.1	2.9	3.0
including				
Road accidents	2.8	3.0	2.9	3.2
Accidents of daily life	1.6	1.5	3.4	3.3
Suicide	3.1	3.0	2.8	2.8
Respiratory disease	2.2	2.3	2.6	2.6
Cirrhosis, alcoholic psychosis	3.0	3.0	2.7	2.7
AIDS	3.9	5.9	3.8	6.3

a. Cancer of the upper airways and digestive tract (including oesophagus).
Source: Inserm SC8.

Table 9 **Variation in "avoidable"[a] mortality rate between 1991 and 1996**
(number of deaths and comparative mortality rates per 100,000 standardised by age, France, both sexes, 1990)

	"Avoidable" mortality related to risk behaviours		"Avoidable" mortality related to care and screening system	
	Men	Women	Men	Women
Number of deaths 1996	27,725	6,400	13,544	10,269
Mortality rate 1996	113.3	25.7	56.5	41.4
Variation 1991-1996[a]	– 22%	– 21%	– 13%	– 11%

a. 1991-1996 variation = (1996 rate – 1991 rate)/1991 rate x 100.
Source: Inserm SC8.

– "avoidable" deaths linked to the medical care system; causes of death whose incidence could be reduced thanks to better management by the medical care system (including screening programmes), possibly reinforced by measures to influence individual behaviours; this selection includes ischaemic heart disease, cerebrovascular and hypertensive diseases, breast cancer, cancer of the uterus, gastric ulcer, appendicitis, abdominal hernia, maternal mortality and perinatal mortality (less than one week).

In men, "avoidable" mortality linked to risk behaviours is 4 times greater than that linked to the medical care system. In contrast, it is "avoidable" mortality linked to the medical care system which occurs more frequently in women (especially cancers of the breast and uterus).

Between 1991 and 1996, a marked decrease in "avoidable" mortality linked to risk behaviours has been noted for both sexes, whereas there has been a far less pronounced decrease in "avoidable" mortality linked to the medical care system.

The age limit used in defining "premature" mortality (65 years) and the distinction made between "avoidable" mortality linked to risk behaviours and "avoidable" mortality related to the medical care system are the indicators usually adopted. These indicators may seem arbitrary, yet they have proved to be of great practical use, particularly in analysing the determinants of inequalities.

Disparities in mortality

Persistent major differences in mortality among different socioprofessional categories

As in most countries, there are wide differences in mortality among the various socioprofessional categories (SPC) in France. Moreover, a recent European study[3] showed that the differences are wider in France than in most European countries. The risk of mortality among men aged 35 to 60 years varies from 10% for management to 20% for manual workers[4]. The most favoured categories are primary and secondary school teachers, engineers, and executives. The most vulnerable are farm and manual workers, and service personnel. These disparities affect both sexes but are far less marked among women. At the family level, the SPC of the husband strongly influences his wife's and children's mortality risk. These differences in mortality tend to lessen with age.

Similar trends in differences have been noted for most causes of death. The greatest inequalities between SPCs are observed for alcohol-related diseases (10 times higher risk of death among men in the category "management, professions" than those in the "manual workers, employees" category in terms of cirrhosis and cancers of the UADT) and, in general, but to a lesser extent, for all diseases linked to risk behaviours (lung cancer, accidents, suicides...).

---

3. Kunst A.E., *Cross-national comparisons of socio-economic differences in mortality*, Rotterdam-Erasmus University, 1997.
4. Desplanques G., *"Les cadres vivent plus vieux"* (Executives live longer), INSEE Première 1991, 158.

An analysis of changes in disparities between the various SPCs over the course of time raises a certain number of methodological problems. However, the studies most recently carried out (covering changes between 1980 and 1991) appear to indicate that inequalities are tending to increase since the risk of death is showing a greater decrease for executives and those in liberal professions than for other categories. The study on variations in life expectancy between 1980 and 1991 differentiated three SPCs ("senior management, the professions", "technicians, employees, owners of retail outlets" and "manual workers") and showed that, regardless of the category considered, there was a general decrease in the risk of death for those aged 35 to 59. However, the gap between the extreme categories increased, basically because of a greater reduction in the risk of death among the elderly in the higher category. In 1991, the life expectancy of 35-year-olds in the "senior management, the professions" category was 8 years longer than that of manual workers of the same age.

Calculations of life expectancy with unimpaired health (LEUH) as a function of SPC show that between 1980 and 1991, the LEUH rose for all SPCs and that the increases were greater than those noted for the corresponding life expectancies[5]. This indicates that, irrespective of the SPC considered, the extra years of life were not achieved at the expense of greater disability. However, the calculations also revealed a parallel accumulation of inequalities since the privileged categories had both a longer life expectancy and fewer disabilities (resulting in a longer LEUH). Over the period studied, the inequalities in LEUH showed a tendency to become even more pronounced among the elderly in the different SPCs.

These results must be interpreted with care, given the complex methodological problems linked to calculations of LEUH by SPC, but they indicate that in overall terms inequalities in mortality and disability accumulate and disadvantage the least favoured SPCs. However, these observed trends refer to the 1980s and no current data are available concerning changes since the beginning of the 1990s.

---

5. Cambois E., *Social inequalities in health expectancies: calculation of health expectancies according to socio-economic status in France*, 10th REVES meeting, Tokyo, October 1997, p. 13.

Part two — Changes in health status

General mortality is decreasing in most regions but the difference between extreme regions remains constant

Since 1991, the general mortality rate has gone down in most regions in France. The only exceptions relate to the regions Pays-de-la-Loire (for both sexes) and Upper Normandy (for men) where slight increases have been noted. The regions in which mortality has shown the greatest decrease are Île-de-France (for both sexes), Limousin (for men) and Nord-Pas-de-Calais, Auvergne, Languedoc-Roussillon, Paca and Corsica (for women).

Considering broad groups of diseases (figure 3), the following exceptions to the general decrease were noted: Picardy (cardiovascular diseases in men); Pays-de-la-Loire (cancers in men); numerous regions, especially western France (cancers in women); Aquitaine, Pays-de-la-Loire and Champagne-Ardenne (violent deaths among men) and Centre, Lorraine and Franche-Comté (violent deaths among women). It should be noted, however, that all the increases were generally very modest.

The differences in mortality between extreme regions showed little change between 1991 and 1996 as far as most diseases are concerned (table 10), the only exceptions being AIDS, carcinoma of the stomach and alcoholism, where the disparities have tended to decrease.

Analyses based on data aggregates showed that the socio-economic characteristics of the populations carried the greatest weight as explanatory factors for inter-regional differences in mortality.

Table 10 **Excess mortality between extreme regions (1996 and 1991)**
(ratio of mortality rates standardised by age, per 100,000, except for Corsica)

	Men		Women	
	1996	1991	1996	1991
All causes	1.4	1.4	1.3	1.2
AIDS	9.8	14.7	11.7	11.7
Cirrhosis, alcoholic cirrhosis	2.9	3.1	4.3	4.7
Cancer of the UADT[a]	2.8	2,9	2.2	2.5
Suicide[b]	2.2	2.3	1.9	2.2
Road accidents[b]	2.1	2.2	2.0	2.1
Lung cancer	2.0	1.9	2.1	2.1
Stomach carcinoma	1.8	2.2	2.0	2.3
Stroke	1.7	1.7	1.6	1.6
Ischaemic heart disease	1.6	1.5	1.7	1.6
Uterine cancer			1.7	1.4
Breast cancer			1.6	1.4
Intestinal cancer	1.5	1.6	1.4	1.5
Accidents of daily life[b]	1.5	1.6	1.4	1.4

a. Cancer of the upper airways and digestive tract (including oesophagus).
b. Except the Île-de-France region.
Source: Inserm SC8.

Indicators of health status

Figure 3 **Variation in regional comparative mortality rates 1991-1996**

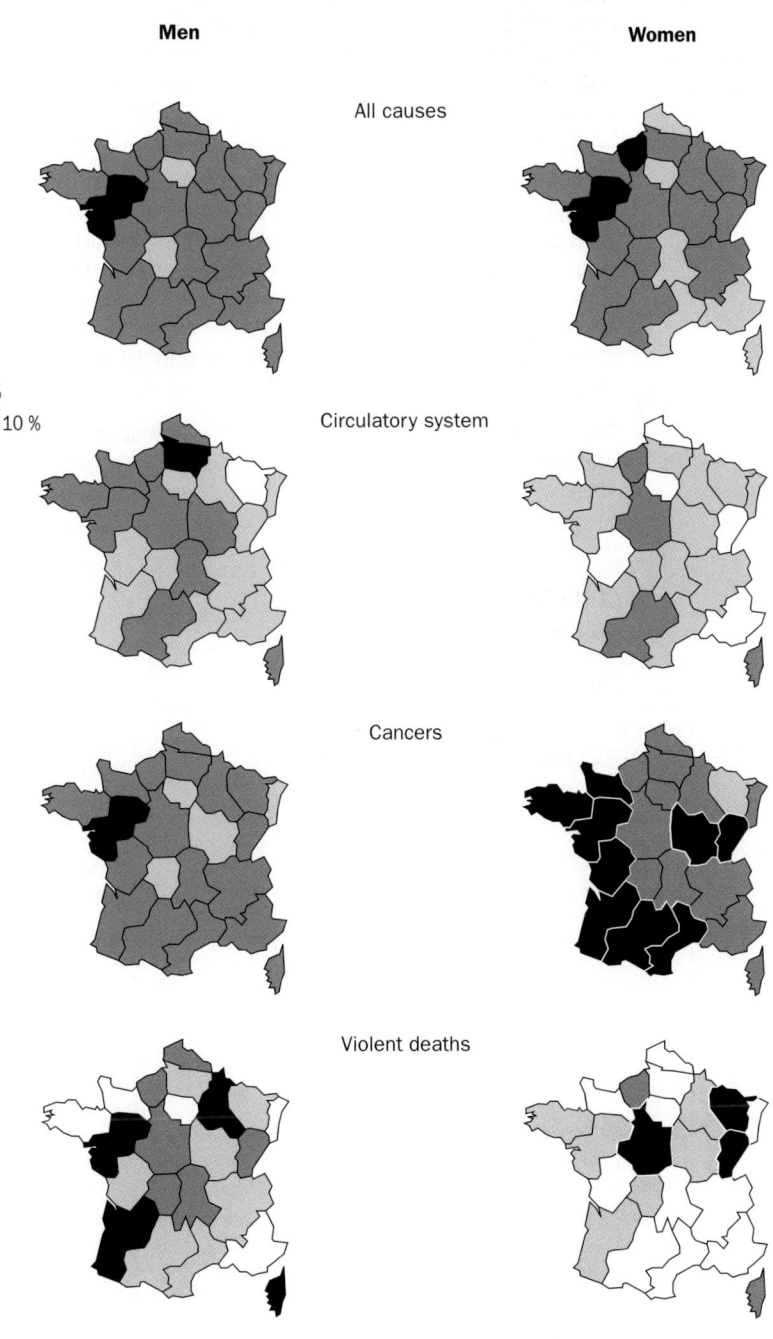

Variation 1991-1995
- increase
- decrease of 0 to -5 %
- decrease of -5 to -10 %
- decrease of more than 10 %

Source: Inserm SC8.

Part two   Changes in health status

In 1996, regardless of sex, Nord-Pas-de-Calais remained the region with the highest general mortality in France (figure 4). It was followed by Brittany and Alsace (for men) and Alsace and Picardy (for women).

The Nord-Pas-de-Calais region topped the list for many conditions (table 11); among men, it had the highest mortality rate for lung cancer, cancers of the UADT, infarction and alcoholism, took second place in terms of intestinal cancer and third place for strokes; among women, it had the highest rate for cancers of the UADT, intestinal cancer, breast cancer and alcoholism, took second place for diseases of the circulatory system and third place for accidents of daily life. The mortality rate is particularly high in Alsace, irrespective of sex, in terms of circulation disorders, for intestinal cancer among men and for cancer of the uterus among women.

The incidence of specific diseases is higher in other regions: Brittany and Normandy for suicide and carcinoma of the stomach,

Table 11   **Regions of maximum mortality according to the cause of death (1992-1994) and sex**
(rates standardised by age, per 100,000)

	Men			Women		
	1	2	3	1	2	3
All causes	NPDC	Brittany	Alsace	NPDC	Alsace	Picardy
Cancer						
Lung cancer	NPDC	Corsica	Lorraine	Corsica	Île-de-France	Lorraine
Cancer of the UADT[a]	NPDC	Brittany	Picardy	NPDC	Upper Normandy	Île-de-France
Intestinal cancer	Alsace	NPDC	Lorraine	NPDC	Lorraine	Picardy
Stomach carcinoma	Upper Normandy	Brittany	Lower Normandy	Upper Normandy	Brittany	Lower Normandy
Melanoma	Alsace	Pays-de-la-Loire	Midi-Pyrénées	Brittany	Picardy	Pays-de-la-Loire
Breast cancer				NPDC	Upper Normandy	Île-de-France
Uterine cancer				Alsace	Picardy	Upper Normandy
Cardiovascular						
Ischaemic heart dis.	NPDC	Alsace	Lower Normandy	Alsace	NPDC	Picardy
Stroke	Alsace	Corsica	NPDC	Corsica	NPDC	Alsace
Cirrhosis, alc. psych.	NPDC	Upper Normandy	Brittany	NPDC	Upper Normandy	Picardy
AIDS	Île-de-France	Paca	L^{oc}-Roussillon	Paca	Île-de-France	Corsica
Violent death						
Road accidents	Corsica	L^{oc}-Roussillon	Picardy	Centre	Corsica	Picardy
Accidents daily life	Brittany	Auvergne	Alsace	Brittany	Burgundy	NPDC
Suicides	Brittany	Lower Normandy	Upper Normandy	Upper Normandy	Brittany	Lower Normandy

a. Cancer of the upper airways and digestive tract (including oesophagus).
Source: Inserm SC8.

Indicators of health status

Figure 4 **Regional comparative mortality rates in 1995 compared with the national mean**

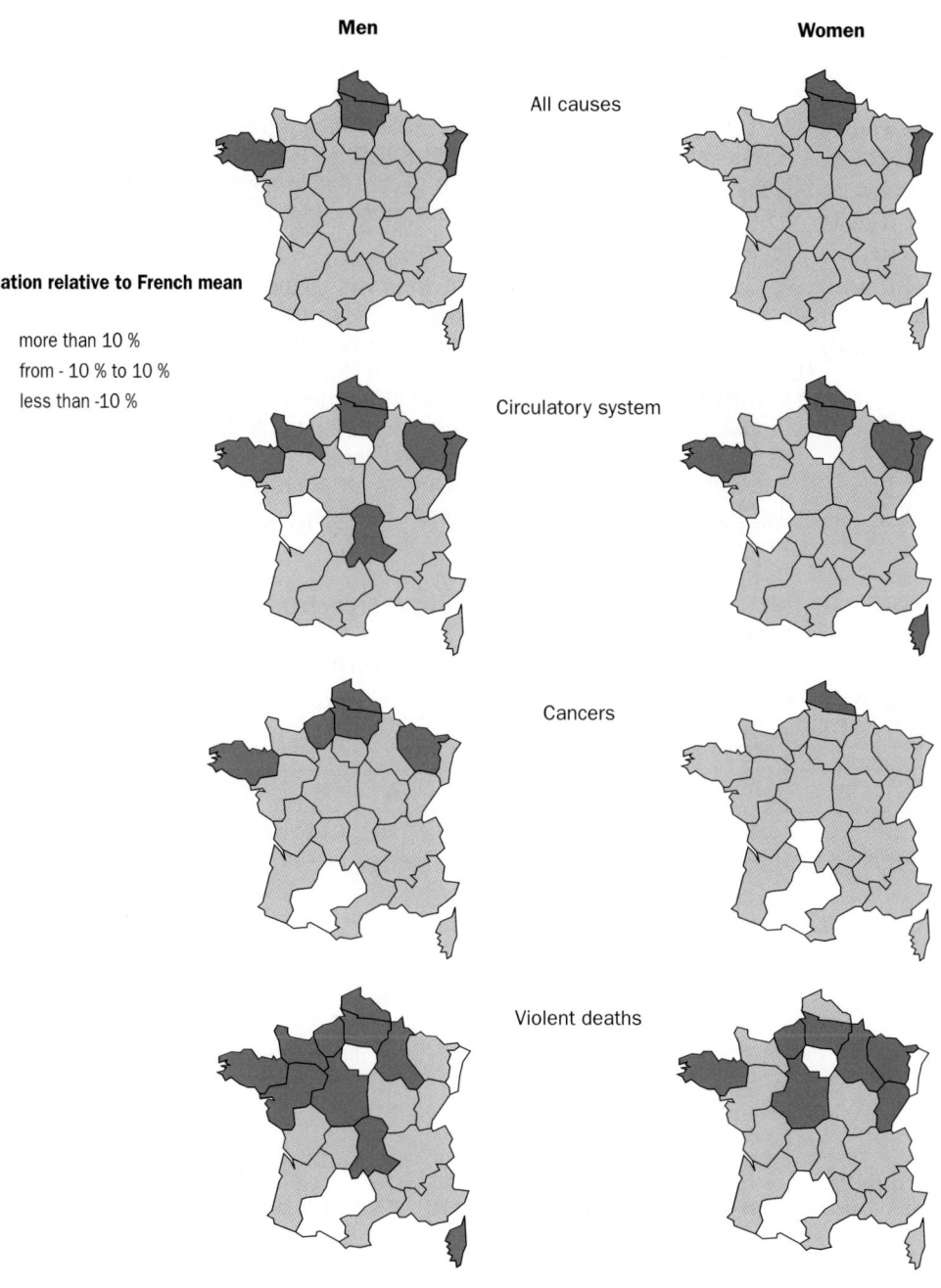

Variation relative to French mean
- more than 10 %
- from -10 % to 10 %
- less than -10 %

Source: Inserm SC8.

Part two Changes in health status

Brittany for accidents of daily life, Corsica for lung cancer, strokes and road accidents, Île-de-France and Paca for AIDS.

The greatest inter-regional differences in mortality were noted for the following diseases: AIDS, alcoholism and cancers of the upper airways and digestive tract (table 11).

General mortality in French overseas territories is similar to that in France (although higher on Réunion Island)

In 1995, 2,479 deaths were recorded in Guadeloupe, 2,340 in Martinique, 558 in Guyana, and 3,488 on Réunion Island. Relative to France, the mortality rate was lower in Martinique, slightly higher in Guadeloupe and Guyana, and markedly higher on Réunion Island (table 12).

In Guadeloupe, Martinique and Réunion Island, diseases of the circulatory system are the prime cause of death, accounting for approximately one third of all deaths. The other causes are cancer (one death in five), followed by violent deaths (one death in 10). In Guyana, there is an appreciable difference in the burden of the respective diseases, with injuries and infectious diseases being more lethal than in the French West Indies and Réunion Island. Although cardiovascular mortality is still predominant, violent death takes second place, ahead of cancer.

Table 12 **Mortality rates standardised by age, French overseas territories, 1995**
(rate per 100,000 inhabitants, both sexes, 1990, decennial age group)

	Guadeloupe		Martinique		Guyana		Réunion		Métropole	
	M	W	M	W	M	W	M	W	M	W
All causes	1,192	731	1,080	645	1,210	720	1,510	872	1,186	676
Cardiovascular disease	369	293	364	249	352	285	521	360	361	234
including										
Infarction	43	38	55	34	19	24	117	74	114	55
Cerebrovascular disease	144	121	139	87	145	117	169	131	85	65
Cancer	257	144	258	134	265	80	336	139	362	166
including										
Lung	22	4	17	4	48	6	69	4	79	11
UADT[a]	36	5	31	5	47	5	50	6	40	5
Stomach	23	15	25	14	18	0	30	10	15	6
Intestine	5	10	16	18	30	6	11	11	37	22
Prostate	87		75		35		56		44	
Breast		13		15		24		17		32
Uterus		23		13		10		20		9
Violent death	138	40	87	34	153	48	128	42	106	50
Respiratory disease	89	36	78	48	66	42	156	85	99	48
Alcoholism and cirrhosis	63	9	37	7	17	13	79	28	29	10
AIDS	28	8	21	4	30	31	5	2	13	3

a. Cancer of the upper airways and digestive tract (including oesophagus).
Source: Inserm SC8.

Indicators of health status

Cardiovascular mortality is about the same in the French West Indies as in France, but is markedly higher on Réunion Island for both sexes. One notable feature is the particularly high incidence of cerebrovascular disease relative to infarction.

Cancer-related mortality is lower in French overseas territories. Some specific differences may be highlighted with regard to location: in French overseas territories, the risk of death due to carcinoma of the stomach is higher, whereas it is lower for intestinal cancer; the incidence of cancer of the uterus is higher whereas it is lower for breast cancer, which is more frequent in France; prostate cancer is the cancer which ravages the greatest number of victims in the French West Indies. Guyana is the territory most affected by violent death (Martinique has the lowest mortality in this respect). Alcohol-related mortality is particularly high on Réunion Island. Lastly, AIDS-related deaths are markedly higher in French overseas territories (apart from Réunion Island) than in France, the highest incidence being noted in Guyana.

Between 1990 and 1995, the mortality rate showed a greater decrease in Guyana than in French West Indian territories, while it remained stable on Réunion Island (table 13). Mortality showed a slight increase among 25-34-year-olds in Guadeloupe. In Martinique, mortality rates increased among those in the 35-44 age group and the very elderly. Unlike Guadeloupe, Martinique did not record any appreciable drop in infantile mortality. In Guyana, there was an almost general reduction in mortality, except among the very young and very old.

Table 13 **Variation in mortality rates standardised by age[a], French overseas territories, 1990 to 1995**

	Guadeloupe		Martinique		Guyana		Réunion	
	M	W	M	W	M	W	M	W
Cardiovascular disease	– 5%	– 3%	– 2%	– 11%	– 25%	– 29%	– 4%	– 7%
Cancer	– 13%	0%	– 4%	– 4%	38%		23%	14%
Violent death	– 1%	– 4%	– 2%	– 8%	– 20%		– 2%	– 8%
Respiratory disease	7%	1%	17%	17%			– 15%	12%
All causes combined	– 8%	– 3%	– 3%	– 9%	– 16%	– 22%	– 1%	0%

The percentage variation was not calculated when fewer than 30 deaths were involved.
a. 1990-1996 variation = (1996 rate – 1990 rate)/1990 rate x 100.
Source: Inserm SC8.

A study of broad groups of diseases showed that there was a decrease in cancer-related mortality and an increase in mortality related to respiratory disease among men in Guadeloupe. In Martinique, the incidence of death due to cardiovascular disease, cancer and violence decreased in all cases but the risk related to respiratory disease increased. The fall in cardiovascular mortality was more conspicuous among women. In Guyana, the reduction in general mortality was primarily due to a lower risk of cardiovascular disease and violent death (on the other hand, increased mortality due to cancer was noted among men). On Réunion Island, cancer-related mortality rose for both sexes (lung and prostate cancer among men, uterus and breast cancer among women). Mortality due to respiratory disease fell in men and rose in women. Lastly, mortality related to alcohol abuse showed a marked reduction in this territory.

These data relate to recorded deaths and not to the deaths of residents (as in France). Only deaths which occurred in the four territories were taken into account (including the deaths of those who were non residents). The deaths of subjects living in French overseas territories but which occurred in France cannot be included in this statistic, thereby limiting its reliability in terms of the causes of death in French overseas territories.

Longest life expectancy for women compared with other European countries but average for men

The maximum difference in life expectancy between men and women in countries belonging to the European Community is noted in France (8 years *versus* 5 in countries such as the United Kingdom, Sweden, Denmark, Iceland and Greece). This difference results in a very dissimilar position in terms of life expectancy among men and women compared with other European countries (table 14), *i.e.* average for French men, and the highest for French women. Between 1991 and 1996, gains in life expectancy were noted for all European countries, although the magnitude of such gains varied for each individual country. France was characterized by an average progression (1.1 year among men and 0.8 year among women). The most marked gains were noted among men

Table 14 **Life expectancy at birth in various European countries (1996 and 1991)**

	Men			Women			Difference women-men	
	1996	1991	Gain[a]	1996	1991	Gain[a]	1996	1991
Germany	73.3	72.2	1.1	79.8	78.7	1.1	6.5	6.5
Spain	74.4	73.4	1.0	81.6	80.6	1.0	7.2	7.2
France	74.0	72.9	1.1	81.9	81.1	0.8	7.9	8.2
Italy	74.9	73.6	1.3	81.3	80.2	1.1	6.4	6.6
Netherlands	74.7	74.0	0.7	80.3	80.1	0.2	5.6	6.1
Portugal	71.0	70.2	0.8	78.5	77.4	1.1	7.5	7.2
United Kingdom	74.4	73.2	1.2	79.3	78.6	0.7	4.9	5.4
Sweden	76.5	74.9	1.6	81.5	80.5	1.0	5.0	5.6

a. Gain in years between 1991 and 1996
Source: Eurostat.

Indicators of health status

living in Finland, Iceland, Sweden, Switzerland and Austria, with fewer gains among women (0.9 year on average for all countries combined and 0.8 year for France). The gap between women and men remained relatively stable between 1990 and 1996 in most countries (slight decrease in France).

France is characterised by a higher risk of death in terms of "premature" mortality and lower in terms of the elderly

When the mortality rates in France are compared with those in other similarly developed countries, a quite remarkable general tendency can be observed. The risk of death is generally markedly higher among the young (especially young men) in France whereas the situation is reversed among the elderly. In particular, the risk of death among men in the 25 to 44 age group is twice as high in France as in countries such as the United Kingdom, Holland or Sweden (similar differences are also noted in many other countries). In contrast, the privileged situation of the French population where the risk of death among the elderly is concerned becomes clearly evident when comparisons are made of life expectancy in the various European countries for persons still alive at age 65 (life expectancy at 65 years). France is then in the leading group of countries in terms of men as well as women (table 15). Since the beginning of the 1990s, many countries have seen a greater decrease in the risk of death in those under 65 than in those over 65.

In order to demonstrate the causes of death which would explain the specific nature of the situation in France (especially where excess "premature" mortality is concerned), the disparities that exist between the risk of death in France and those in England and Wales combined[6] may be taken as an example.

Table 15 **Life expectancy at 65 years in various European countries (1995 and 1991)**

	Men			Women			Difference women-men	
	1995	1991	Gain[a]	1995	1991	Gain[a]	1995	1991
Germany	14.7	14.2	0.5	18.5	17.8	0.7	3.8	3.6
Spain		15.6			19.2			3.6
France	16.1	15.7	0.4	20.6	20.1	0.5	4.5	4.4
Italy		15.1			18.9			3.8
Netherlands	14.7	14.5	0.2	19.1	19.0	0.1	4.4	4.5
Portugal	14.3	14.0	0.3	17.7	17.2	0.5	3.4	3.2
United Kingdom	14.6	14.2	0.4	18.1	17.8	0.3	3.5	3.6
Sweden	16.0	15.4	0.6	19.7	19.2	0.5	3.7	3.8

a. Gain in years between 1991 and 1995
Source: Eurostat.

---

6. Jougla E., Le Toullec A. Les causes de la surmortalité en France, comparaison avec la situation en Angleterre-Galles, *Concours Médical*, 1998 (à paraître).

Overall, the comparative mortality rates due to all causes combined for the entire population are lower in France. Since the start of the 1980s, the risk of death has dropped sharply in both countries. However, the reduced risk has not been the same in all age brackets. A notable drop in the mortality rate, similar in extent, was observed among the youngest section of the population in both countries. Less risk reduction occurred in the 25 to 44 age group, while the decrease was greater in England-and-Wales among those aged 45 to 64. On the other hand, greater progress was recorded among the elderly in France. These changes resulted in a widening of the mortality gap between the two countries among those under 65 (augmentation in excess mortality, especially among men, in France), whereas mortality differences remained relatively constant in those over 65 (excess mortality in England-and-Wales).

The differences in mortality in the two countries depended on the type of condition studied (tables 16 and 17).

The risk of death due to the following causes was markedly higher in France: AIDS (risk multiplied by a factor of more than 5), suicide (risk multiplied by 3), alcoholism (risk multiplied by 3 among men and by 2 among women), road accidents (risk multiplied by 3 in those under 65), other types of accident (those over 45), cancers of the UADT among 25-64-year-old men and lung cancer (in men aged 25 to 44 years). There was no appreciable difference in the degree of excess mortality in France and England-and-Wales for the majority of these causes as a function of age; however, since the type of cause had a greater influence on mortality among the young, the increased incidence of the causes led to the overall excess mortality noted among young adults in France compared with England-and-Wales.

There were fewer causes of excess mortality in England-and-Wales: infarction (risk multiplied by 3 in those over 45), diseases of the respiratory system (over 45s) and, only among women, lung cancer in those over 45 and cancers of the UADT in those over 65.

It is also of interest to analyse the relative weight of the various causes that account for excess "premature" mortality among males in France compared to England-and-Wales (table 18). The relative weight is based on the degree of excess mortality arising from any given cause and the total number of deaths resulting from the cause in question. The incidence of road accidents (40% of general excess mortality) essentially explains the general excess mortality in France among those under 25. Among those in the 25 to 44 age group, three types of disease are responsible for 60% of the excess mortality: AIDS, suicide and road accidents. Between 45 and 64 years, cancers of the UADT, alcoholism and lung cancer account for half the excess mortality noted in France.

Indicators of health status

Table 16 **Causes of death for which the risk of death in France was more than twice that in England-and-Wales in 1993, as a function of sex and age**

	Under 25 years		25-44 years		45-64 years		65 years and over	
	Cause	Rate[a]	Cause	Rate[a]	Cause	Rate[a]	Cause	Rate[a]
Men	Road acc.[d]	2.5	AIDS	7.6	AIDS	6.3	Suicide	5.5
			C. UADT[b]	3.9	Alcohol[c]	4.6	Alcohol[c]	4.8
			Road acc.[d]	3.2	C. UADT[b]	3.2	Other acc.[e]	3.4
			Alcohol[c]	3.1	Road acc.[d]	3.0	Road acc.[d]	2.1
			Lung c.[f]	2.7	Other acc.[e]	2.9		
			Suicide	2.6	Suicide	2.8		
Women	Road acc.[d]	2.7	AIDS	14.3	AIDS	12.6	Suicide	4.8
	Suicide	2.7	Suicide	3.6	Suicide	3.9	Other acc.[e]	3.1
			Road acc.[d]	3.4	Road acc.[d]	3.1	Alcohol[c]	2.6
			Alcohol[c]	2.3	Alcohol[c]	3.0		
					Other acc.[e]	2.0		

a. Ratio of "French mortality rate/English mortality rate" (comparative rates).
b. Cancer of the upper airways and digestive tract (including oesophagus).
c. Cirrhosis and alcoholic psychosis.
d. Road accidents.
e. Other types of accident.
f. Lung cancer.
Source: Inserm SC8.

Table 17 **Causes of death for which the risk of death in England-and-Wales was more than twice that in France in 1993, as a function of sex and age**

	Under 25 years		25-44 years		45-64 years		65 and over	
	Cause	Rate[a]	Cause	Rate[a]	Cause	Rate[a]	Cause	Rate[a]
Men					Infarction	3.5	Infarction	3.2
							Resp. system[c]	2.4
Women			Infarction	2.8	Infarction	5.3	Lung c.[d]	4.0
					Resp. system[c]	3.1	Infarction	3.3
					Lung c.[d]	3.1	Resp. system[c]	2.9
					CVA[e]	2.0	C. UADT[b]	2.8

a. Ratio of "French mortality rate/English mortality rate" (comparative rates).
b. Cancer of the upper airways and digestive tract (including oesophagus).
c. Diseases of the respiratory system.
d. Lung cancer.
e. Cerebrovascular accident (stroke).
Source: Inserm SC8.

Table 18 **Weight of various causes that account for the excess premature mortality observed among men in France relative to England-and-Wales in 1993, as a function of age**

Under 25 years		25-44 years		45-64 years	
Road accidents	41%	AIDS	23%	Cancer of UADT[a]	19%
Suicide	12%	Suicide	20%	Alcoholism[b]	17%
Other accidents	6%	Road accidents	16%	Lung cancer	11%
Other diseases	5%	Alcoholism[b]	7%	Other cancers	15%
Ill defined causes	35%	Other accidents	5%	Suicide	8%
		Cancer of UADT[a]	4%	Other accidents	8%
		Lung cancer	4%	Road accidents	4%
		Other diseases	5%	AIDS	4%
		Ill defined causes	15%	Other diseases	4%
				Ill defined causes	11%
Total	100%	Total	100%	Total	100%

Reading: 23% of the general excess mortality among men aged 25-44 years in France relative to England-and-Wales is due to the higher frequency of AIDS-related death in France.
a. Cancer of the upper airways and digestive tract (including oesophagus).
b. Cirrhosis and alcoholic psychosis.
Source: Inserm SC8.

For some of these causes (cancers of the UADT, alcoholism, other accidents), premature mortality rates among men have shown a greater decrease since the 1980s in France, although their current level still remains much higher in France. Changes over time in many other causes have not been to France's advantage (figure 5). The lag has not diminished for road accidents and suicide (the difference between the two countries has even tended to widen). As for lung cancer in men under 65, the tendency has even reversed (rates are currently higher in France whereas the opposite was true at the beginning of the 1980s). As for diseases carrying a higher risk of death in England-and-Wales, the differences between the two countries have shown a tendency to shrink (infarction and diseases of the respiratory system), although the mortality rates are still higher in England-and-Wales.

The causes of death responsible for excess "premature" mortality in France are very specific in terms of public health and all are highly related to subjective behaviour and lifestyle: alcoholism (psychosis, cirrhosis, cancers of the UADT, accidents), smoking (lung cancer, cancers of the UADT, etc.), risk-taking (road accidents, other types of accident, etc.), sexual behaviour (AIDS), etc.. Since these types of disease are predominantly responsible for death among the young, their high incidence gives rise to general excess premature mortality in France. Over the age of 65, most of these same causes still carry a much increased risk in France but, since the diseases are less influential in terms of mortality among the elderly, they no longer lead to general excess mortality.

Indicators of health status

Figure 5 **Variations in the mortality rates of men under 65 in France and England-and-Wales (1980-1993)**

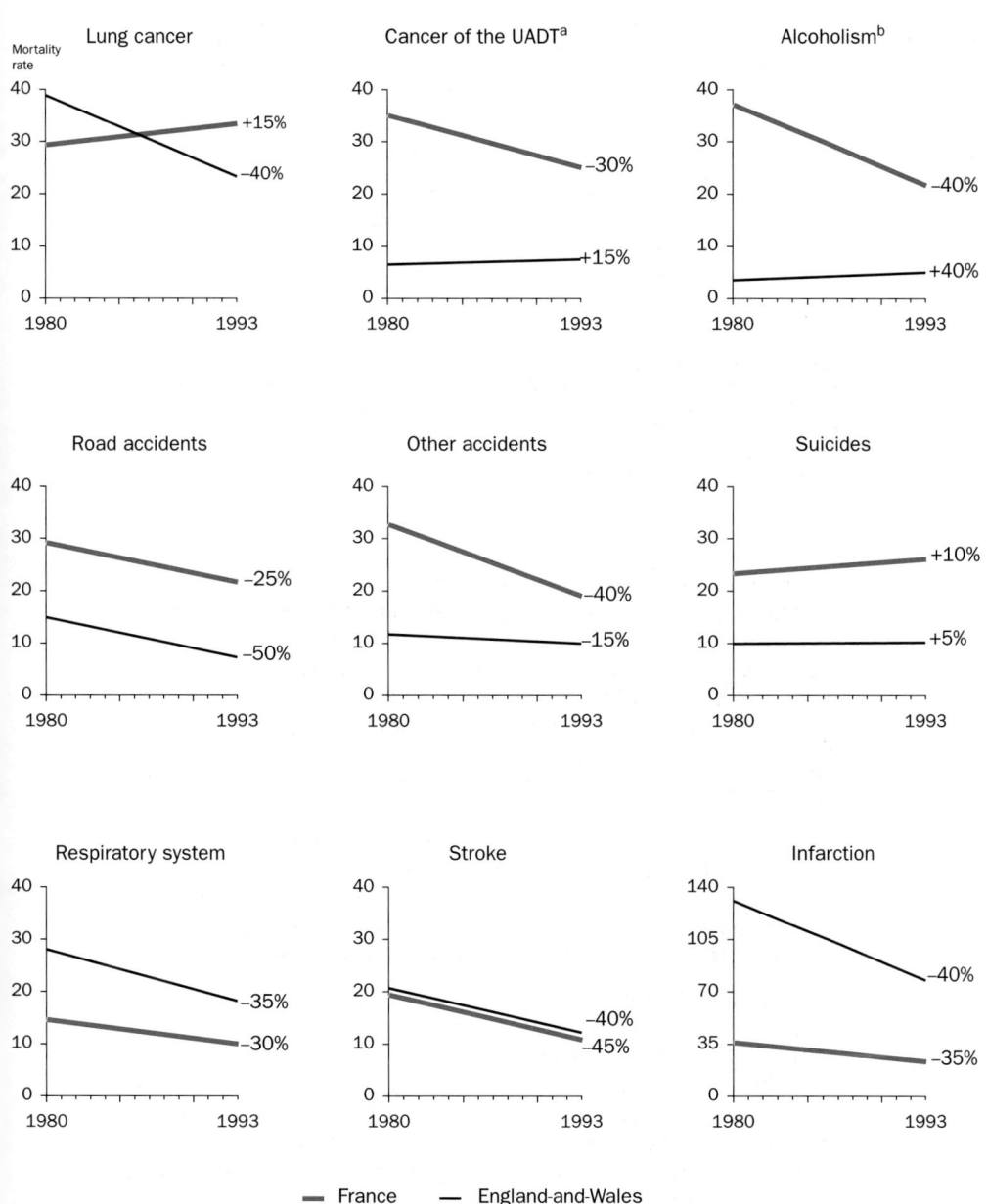

a. Cancers of the upper airways and digestive tract (including the oesophagus).
b. Cirrhosis and alcoholic psychosis.

Source: Inserm SC8.

On the other hand, the incidence of circulation disorders is far higher in England-and-Wales than in France and leads to general excess mortality in England-and-Wales in those over 65.

The trends described not only hold true for the comparison of France with England-and-Wales but are also observed when France is compared with numerous other countries.

Morbidity

How to measure morbidity in the population?

The measurement of morbidity, *i.e.* the incidence of illness, comes up against two major difficulties[7]. The first is the very concept of disease: it is usually a complex exercise to define what illness is, when it begins, and when it can be considered to be over. The second difficulty lies in defining the field studied. A knowledge of "actual" morbidity, quite independent of the subject and medical care system, is a theoretical concept – it is generally easier to note the morbidity stated by individuals themselves or diagnosed by doctors during a medical examination or request for medical attention.

There is no source in France which would give an overall view of actual morbidity. Measurements have been made of the prevalence or incidence of a certain number of specific diseases but they fail to cover either an entire area of disease or even, frequently, the entire population.

Thus, registers of disease make it possible to estimate the incidence of diseases such as cancer or myocardial infarction which can, to a certain extent, be diagnosed regardless of individual subjectivity or fluctuations in requests for medical attention, at the cost of special efforts made in defined geographic regions. The results concerning incidence obtained from these disease registers during the first ten years are given in the description of health indicators.

The only global approaches available provide a knowledge of (i) morbidity as stated by individuals and (ii) the reasons for medical care consumption, especially the reasons for seeking treatment by a doctor.

"Stated" morbidity constitutes the sub-set of diseases that individuals are willing to declare during a survey. It is therefore only a partial view of an individual's disease since it suffers from unintentional or deliberate omissions by the person making the declaration. It reflects the knowledge that individuals have of their own health status, particularly when acquired through contacts

---

7. Sermet C., *"De quoi souffre-t-on? Description et évolution de la morbidité déclarée 1980-1991"* (What ails us? Description and variation in declared morbidity 1980-1991), Solidarité-Santé N°. 1-1994, pp. 37-56.

Indicators of health status

with the medical profession. In one way, stated morbidity may therefore be regarded as dependent on an individual's consumption of medical care.

Variation in stated morbidity reflects two main factors: the actual prevalence of diseases, and changes in the declarations. It is not necessarily directly correlated with the variation in actual morbidity. The first of these factors, the actual prevalence of diseases, can change as a result of variations in the incidence of the diseases, leading to an increase or decline in the number of new cases, and/or a modification in the duration of the disease or in patient survival.

DEFINITIONS

Prevalence: the number of cases of a given disease or persons suffering from the disease, existing in a specific population at a given time, regardless of the date of onset of the disease.

Incidence: the number of new cases of a given disease or persons suffering from the disease, in a given period, in a specific population.

Moreover, a progression in the majority of known factors contributes to an improvement in the declarations:
– better circulation of medical information to individuals,
– increased public awareness of specific conditions,
– better methods of collection,
– advances in medical knowledge so that screening of diseases is more efficient,
– treatment innovations justifying more extensive detection of certain conditions,
– increase in requests for medical care so that diseases can be diagnosed more often...

All these factors, together with a growing number of doctors, contribute to the increasing provision of medical care to the population whose individual health concerns assume ever greater importance.

All these factors have played a part in France in the last few years and make it difficult to interpret the increases observed in most declarations of diseases. On the other hand, they add weight to the idea that decreases in stated prevalence may reflect actual declines in morbidity.

As for data concerning the reasons for medical care or seeking medical care, they are derived from surveys of sessions carried out by doctors. The surveys examined the characteristics of the consultations: patients, reasons or diagnoses, prescriptions, etc. In this context, the incidence of diseases noted does not reflect

Part two — Changes in health status

the prevalence of the conditions among the general population for the following two reasons:
– only individuals who consulted a doctor in private practice were included in the surveys,
– the more often a person consults a doctor, the more likely he is to be included in the survey.

Morbidity as stated by the population

Apart from dental and ophthalmological conditions, cardiovascular, respiratory and bone and joint diseases predominate for both sexes.

An analysis of changes in stated morbidity can be made on the basis of two 4-year cycles – 1988 to 1991 and 1992 to 1995 – from annual surveys on health and social protection carried out by CREDES. The results are shown in table 19.

Table 19 **Variation in stated morbidity as a function of major pathologies**
(number of diseases per 100 persons)

	Men		Women	
	1992-1995	Variation 92-95/88-91	1992-1995	Variation 92-95/88-91
Total	292	4%*	360	6%*
Infectious and parasitic diseases	3	16%	4	5%
Cancer	1	ns	2	– 15%
Endocr., nutrition, metab., immune disorders	9	24%	10	37%
Diseases of blood and haematopoietic org.	0	ns	1	ns
Mental disorders	6	45%	10	20%
Diseases of nervous system	4	43%	8	40%
Ophthalmological disorders	56	8%	67	9%
Ear diseases	11	10%	8	10%
Diseases of the circulatory system	28	25%	37	12%
including hypertension	10	25%	11	1%
Diseases of the respiratory system	20	5%	21	7%
Mouth and teeth conditions	78	– 9%	82	– 7%
Diseases solely of the digestive tract	14	– 3%	21	2%
Diseases of urogenital organs	4	23%	13	31%
Complications of pregnancy			0	ns
Diseases of skin and subcutaneous cell tissue	7	0%	10	4%
Musculoskeletal, muscle, connective tissue disorders	20	3%	29	9%
Ill defined signs, symptoms and morbid conditions	13	– 2%	20	– 8%
Traumatic lesions, poisoning	3	– 11%	2	– 4%
Others	12	19%	13	23%

Reading: for the period 1992-1995, 28 diseases of the circulatory system were declared per 100 men. This number is age-adjusted. The French population as of 1 January 1990 served as the reference population. The variations marked with an asterisk(*) indicate a 95% significant difference in the raw data between the two four-year periods.

Source: CREDES surveys on health and social protection 1988-1991 and 1992-1995

For the period 1992-1995, the most frequently stated disorders consisted of dental and ophthalmological conditions. These headings included benign problems such as cavities, myopia, presbyopia, etc. Their recording in terms of stated morbidity is warranted since they frequently entail requests for care from health professionals.

They were followed by diseases of the cardiovascular system which were more frequent among women (37%) than men (28%), basically because of the widespread prevalence of venous conditions among women.

The order of other diseases then varied according to sex. Among men, 20% declared a disease of the respiratory system, 20% a bone and joint disease, and 14% a disease of the gastrointestinal system.

Among women, the following were noted: bone and joint diseases 29%, diseases of the gastrointestinal system 21%, and diseases of the respiratory system 21%.

For both men and women, there was a notable increase in declarations of mental disorders, diseases of the nervous system, the circulatory system, ophthalmological disorders and "other conditions". In addition, there was an increase in declarations of endocrine and metabolic diseases among women, as well as diseases of the urogenital organs and bones and joints. Conversely, a progression in stated infectious and parasitic diseases only occurred in men. Finally, both sexes made fewer declarations of dental conditions in between the two periods.

Under 15-year-olds: dental and visual problems and respiratory conditions predominate

Among the under-15s, the following were predominant: dental problems 25%, diseases of the respiratory system 25%, and ophthalmological problems 20%. These three very frequent groups were followed by diseases of the ear 7%, skin 7%, and gastrointestinal system 5%. The differences between girls and boys were small: declarations of diseases of the respiratory system were slightly more numerous among boys, while visual problems and skin diseases were more frequent among girls.

Thus, for this age group, there are two disease categories, *i.e.* mostly benign disorders affecting the eyes and teeth, myopia, hyperopia, cavities, etc., and acute infectious ORL and respiratory diseases – rhinopharyngitis, otitis, sore throats, etc. (table 20).

16-64 years: onset of age-related conditions

Apart from dental problems noted in 91% of individuals and ophthalmological problems noted in 60%, the most frequent conditions came under the heading of diseases of the circulatory system 24%, the bone and joint system 23%, the respiratory system 19%, and the gastrointestinal system 17%. All these conditions were stated far more frequently by women. Only diseases of the ear and injuries were slightly more frequent among men.

Adults were therefore characterised by the onset of chronic diseases, many of which were age-related: ischaemic heart disease, arterial and venous problems, hypertension, arthritis, disk disease, etc. (table 20).

65 years and over: marked prevalence of cardiovascular and bone and joint diseases

Although ophthalmological problems were still the most frequently stated, disease among the elderly was marked by the predominance of cardiovascular and bone and joint diseases. Cardiovascular diseases were noted 112 times per 100 persons, *i.e.* more than one per person on average, and bone and joint diseases 63 times per 100.

Dental problems were still very frequent, with a prevalence of 105 per 100 persons. Three groups of diseases were more often declared among men: ear conditions, diseases of the respiratory system and urogenital disorders (table 20).

Table 20 **Stated morbidity as a function of major pathologies and age, 1992-1995** (number of diseases per 100 persons)

	Under 15 years	16-64 years	65 and over
Total	**107**	**319**	**548**
Infectious and parasitic diseases	2.8	4	4
Cancer	0.1	2	3
Endocr., nutrition, metab., immune disorders	0.3	8	33
Mental disorders	1.3	9	16
Diseases of nervous system	1.0	8	8
Ophthalmological disorders	20	60	24
Ear diseases	7	6	26
Diseases of the circulatory system	0.3	24	112
Diseases of the respiratory system	25	19	24
Mouth and teeth conditions	25	91	105
Diseases solely of the digestive tract	5	17	39
Diseases of urogenital organs	0.7	10	11
Diseases of skin and subcutaneous cell tissue	7	9	7
Musculosk., muscle, connective tissue disorders	1.5	23	63
Ill defined signs, symptoms and morbid cond.	4.0	16	32
Traumatic lesions, poisoning	1.5	3	4
Others	2.7	10	34

Reading: for the period 1992-1995, 112 diseases of the circulatory system were declared per 100 persons aged 65 and over.
Source: EPPM-IMS France survey

In 8 years, fewer dental problems among children and young adults

The changes noted between the two periods 1988-1991 and 1991-1995 varied as a function of both age and the disease considered. Those declarations which showed an increase are difficult to interpret since most factors that affected them were inclined to cause an increase. Decreases, on the other hand, would seem to indicate actual reductions in the prevalence of disease.

The only significant decreases recorded relate to dental conditions, with an approximately 31% fall in children and 7% in adults: in contrast, they remained stable among the elderly. The reduction among children was primarily related to improved oral and dental prevention and has been confirmed by other sources.

The other significant variations observed were all increases in the frequency of declarations. The most important were, for women over 16: diseases of the circulatory system, mental disorders and ophthalmological problems; for women aged 16 to 64: diseases of the nervous system; and for older women: diseases of the urogenital system.

Four groups of diseases underwent significant increases among men in the same period: cardiovascular, ophthalmological and urogenital diseases, and diseases of the nervous system. In addition, but only among the elderly, endocrine, metabolic and mental disorders and bone and joint conditions showed a substantial increase.

Reasons for consulting doctors in private practice

Between 1991 and 1995, the number of sessions (consultations and visits) carried out by doctors increased by 7.7% according to CNAMTS data. IMS (Intercontinental Medical Statistics) France data revealed an increase of about 12.6%, but the permanent survey of medical prescribing by IMS France covers a more limited field since it only includes doctors who prescribe allopathic medicines in private practice (table 21).

An analysis of the reasons for the sessions showed that the overall structure was stable from 1991 to 1995. The most frequent reasons were diseases of the circulatory system, 26.3 per 100 sessions in 1995-1996, followed by diseases of the respiratory system, 22.1 per 100 sessions. Next came "ill defined signs, symptoms, and morbid conditions", 13.6, mental disorders, 12.7, and bone and joint diseases, 12.5 per 100 sessions.

Overall, the mean number of reasons per 100 sessions rose by 7%. All illness groups were concerned by the increase, to varying extents. The steepest increases were noted for "other reasons" (+ 17%), bone and joint diseases (+ 16%), cancer (+ 14%),

Part two Changes in health status

Table 21 **Variation in reasons for consulting a doctor in private practice, 1992-1996**

	1992		1996		Variation 1992-1996
	N. reasons (thousands)	N. reasons (100 s.)	N. reasons (thousands)	N. reasons (100 s.)	N. reasons (100 s.)
All reasons	450,883	148.4	541,468	158.3	7%*
Infectious and parasitic diseases	19,956	6.6	23,045	6.7	3%
Cancer	4,022	1.3	5,174	1.5	14%*
Endocr, nutri, metab, immune disorders	35,194	8.3	30,477	8.9	7%*
Diseases of blood and haematopoietic org.	1,863	0.6	2,041	0.6	– 2%
Mental disorders	34,494	11.4	43,392	12.7	12%*
Diseases of nervous system	7,341	2.4	8,126	2.4	– 2%*
Ophthalmological disorders	21,164	7.0	23,058	6.7	– 3%*
Ear diseases	8,081	2.7	9,927	2.9	9%*
Diseases of the circulatory system	80,532	26.5	89,920	26.3	– 1%
Diseases of the respiratory system	63,032	20.7	75,692	22.1	7%*
Mouth and teeth conditions	1,869	0.6	2,238	0.7	5%*
Diseases solely of the digestive tract	19,674	6.5	23,068	6.8	4%*
Diseases of urogenital organs	16,832	5.5	21,435	6.3	13%*
Complications of pregnancy	2,258	0.7	2,841	0.8	12%
Diseases of skin and subcutaneous cell tissue	17,399	5.7	19,679	5.8	0%
Musculosk., muscle, connective tissue disorders	32,742	10.8	42,645	12.5	16%*
Congenital conditions	535	0.2	508	0.2	– 17%
Perinatal conditions	418	0.1	480	0.1	0%
Ill defined signs, sympt. and morbid cond.	36,631	12.1	46,343	13.6	12%*
Traumatic lesions, poisoning	13,727	4.5	14,694	4.3	– 5%
Others	43,119	14.2	56,685	16.6	17%*
Total number of sessions	**303,861**		**341,982**		**13%**

Reading: the reason "disease of the circulatory system" was noted 26 times per 100 sessions carried out by a doctor in 1996. Since any given patient could consult for several reasons belonging to the same group of diseases (e.g. varicose veins and hypertension), fewer sessions were actually concerned than is indicated by the number of reasons per 100 sessions. The variations marked with an asterisk (*) indicate a 95% significant difference in the raw data over the four years.

Source: EPPM-IMS France survey

diseases of the urogenital organs (+ 13%), and mental symptoms (+ 12%) and disorders (+ 12%).

These increases were partially related to modifications made in the survey's method of codification. However, the modifications were introduced in December 1995 and do not account for all the changes noted. From 1995 onwards, an increase in requests for medical care was recorded in the case of cancer, diseases of the ear and "other reasons", with a decrease in the case of ophthalmological conditions.

Conclusion Available morbidity data in France show an increase in declarations of numerous types of disease.

However, it is impossible to say to what extent such augmentations are related to an actual rise in the incidence of the diseases or whether they are linked to modifications in the declarations, since all the factors which affect declarations tended to cause an increase. On the other hand, the reduction noted for conditions of the mouth and teeth, principally in children and young adults, is apparently genuine and probably greater in extent than it would seem for the very reason that these factors have boosted declarations.

Finally, there is no overlap between the changes noted in broad areas of disease in terms of disease declarations and the reasons for seeking medical care. The factors influencing one or the other of these indicators are actually different and their effects are hard to compare.

Specific indicators

Accidents of daily life

Accidents of daily life occur at home, in school or during leisure activities and are a prominent cause of mortality and morbidity[8]. They were the cause of 18,000 deaths in 1996 and were responsible for 845,000 admissions to hospital departments providing short-stay medical care during 1993. On the basis of the 1991 decennial survey of health and medical care, it was estimated that a total of 8.4 million accidents of daily life had an effect, however benign, in terms of health in the year considered.

Variation in mortality due to accidents of daily life

Mortality data reveal a slow but regular decline in the number of deaths due to accidents of daily life: 22,846 in 1981, 21,241 in 1986, 19,150 in 1991, then 18,077 in 1996, *i.e.* a drop of about 20% in fifteen years.

However, these crude results take no account of the pattern of mortality resulting from accidents in the course of daily living: such mortality increases exponentially in the elderly and is therefore highly susceptible to ageing among the population.

Table 22 shows that the mortality rate for accidents of daily life in 1995 was lowest in the 5-14 years age bracket (2 per 100,000).

The rate subsequently showed a regular increase with age up to 36 per 100,000 for 65-74-year-olds and then attained values on an altogether different scale for those very advanced in years:

---

[8]. Direction générale de la Santé (National Health Directorate), *"Les accidents de la vie courante"* (Accidents of daily life), Paris, La Documentation Française, 1997, 185 p.

Part two Changes in health status

566 per 100,000 from 85 to 94 years and 1,667 per 100,000 in those 95 and over. So that in 1995, 42% of such accident-related deaths involved persons over 85 and almost two thirds (63%) involved those over 75.

Table 22 **Variation in the number of deaths and mortality rate due to accidents of daily life as a function of age**

	Total	0-1 year	1-4 years	5-14 years	15-24 years	25-34 years	35-44 years	45-54 years	55-64 years	65-74 years	75-84 years	85-94 years	95 years and over
1986													
Number	1,227	271	249	274	831	896	976	1,119	1,521	1,805	5,806	6,504	975
Rate/100,000	38	36	8	4	10	11	13	19	25	49	198	825	2,657
1991													
Number	19,150	209	216	206	622	791	946	914	1,345	1,688	4,552	6,487	1,174
Rate /100,000	34	28	7	3	7	9	11	15	23	37	162	666	2,079
1995													
Number	18,107	92	183	152	492	664	825	959	1,290	1,956	3,813	6,429	1,252
Rate /100,000	31	13	6	2	6	8	10	13	23	38	144	566	1,667

Source: Inserm SC8.

From 1986 to 1995, the mortality rate per 100,000 inhabitants dropped for all age brackets. However, the decrease was particularly marked for the two highest age brackets, i.e. – 32% and – 36%.

The relatively slow decrease in the number of deaths was therefore entirely due to ageing in the population and a very large increase in the number of persons aged 85 and over – this should not be allowed to mask the progress that has been made. In actual fact, the comparative mortality rate, which measures variations on a constant age basis, dropped by 14% between 1991 and 1996: if this trend continues, there will have been a 25% decrease by the year 2000 – i.e. more than the 20% target set in the 1994 report (figure 6). Nevertheless, the stagnation in the comparative rate for both sexes observed in 1995-1996 will have to be checked in the future to make sure the trend has not been interrupted.

Falls and suffocation alone accounted for 72% of the mortality due to accidents of daily life and overwhelmingly concerned the very elderly: in 1995, the initial cause of death was a fall in 5,639 cases and ingestion or suffocation in 1,264 cases among those over 85, i.e. 90% of the mortality due to accidents of daily life at these ages. These two types of accident are still responsible for 80% of deaths in the 75-84 age group.

At present, it is difficult to analyse the specific causes for the spectacular reduction in deaths due to accidents of daily life in

Figure 6 **Mortality due to accidents of daily life (all ages)**
(comparative rates smoothed over 3-year periods)

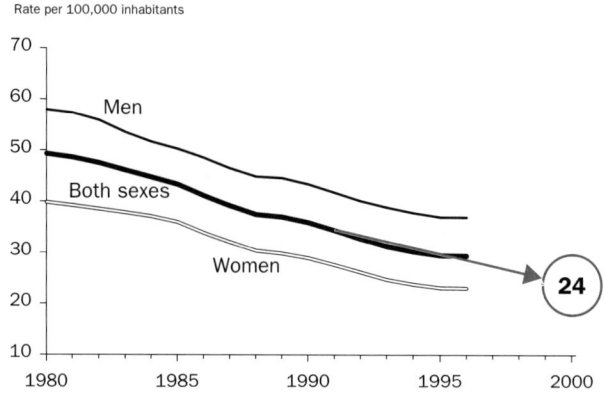

Source: Inserm SC8.

the elderly. Given that epidemiological studies have noted, for a given age and sex, a tendency for the incidence of osteoporotic fractures to increase, then presumably an improvement in the management of accident victims has made a major contribution in prolonging survival.

The numerical importance of deaths due to falls or suffocation in the elderly must not disguise the relative importance of deaths due to accidents of daily life among the young. In fact, they account for one death in five among children aged one to four years, one in eight among those aged five to fourteen years, and one in ten in those between the ages of fifteen and twenty four years.

Morbidity due to accidents of daily life

According to the 1991 decennial survey on health and medical care, the number of accidents of daily life which required at least one request for attention from a doctor or pharmacist was put at about 8.4 million during 1991. Half of these accidents occurred in the home or near vicinity and the other half during leisure or school activities. According to the survey, while 20% of these accidents (1.7 million) were minor in that only pharmaceutical purchases were necessary, three out of five (5.2 million) were sufficiently alarming or serious to generate a visit to a doctor or medical auxiliary, and one in eight (1.5 million) led to an interruption in activity. The survey also showed that the type of accident varied according to sex and age, with domestic accidents preponderant among women, young children and the elderly, leisure-related accidents among men, and leisure- and school-related accidents among adolescents.

Part two Changes in health status

Figure 8 **Variation in the number of killed (at 30 days) per million inhabitants**

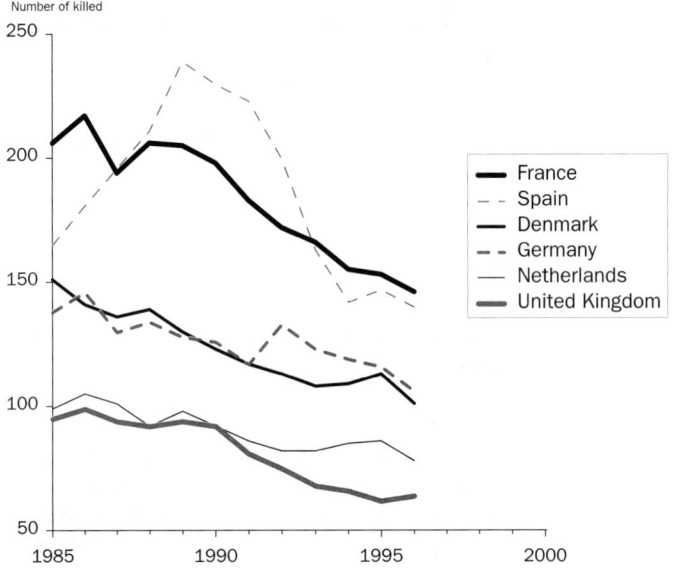

Source: National Interministerial Road Safety Surveillance Agency.

Figure 9 **Mortality due to road accidents (all ages)**
(comparative rates smoothed over 3-year periods)

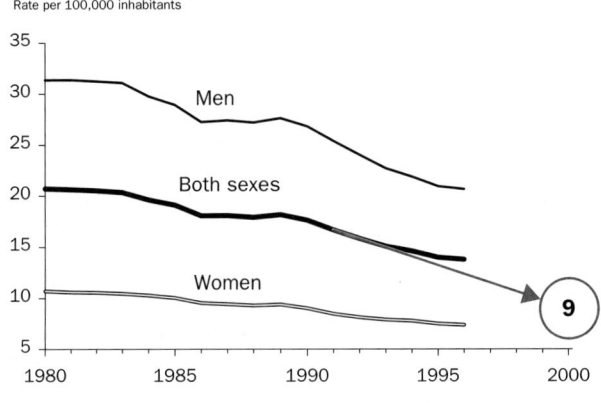

Source: Inserm SC8.

Victims of road accidents in 1997

A breakdown into user categories shows that pedestrians represented 11.3% of the injured and 11.6% of those killed, cyclists 4.1% and 4.2%, users of two-wheeled vehicles (includes drivers and passengers) 22.8% and 16.3%, and users (drivers and passengers) of private vehicles 57.9% and 63.4% respectively. A breakdown of the number of those killed by age group and by user category shows that persons 65 and over accounted for a very large share of pedestrians who were killed (395, *i.e.* 42.5%), while children under 14 represented 10.4% of the total number of pedestrians involved in fatal accidents (97 cases). Among users of two-wheeled vehicles, 493 of those killed were aged 15-24 and represented 37.9% of the total. 15-24-year-olds and 25-44-year-olds accounted for 27.9% and 33.5% respectively of users of private vehicles killed in road accidents.

Overall, it is 15-24-year-olds who were by far the most vulnerable with a mortality rate of 262 per million inhabitants compared with 154 in the case of 25-44-year-olds, 153 for those over 65, 110 for those aged 45-64, and 34 for those under 15. The same is even more true in terms of morbidity since the rate of road accident injury per million inhabitants was 6,682 for those aged 15-24 compared with 3,491 among those aged 25-44, 2,048 for those aged 45-64, 1,508 for the over- 65s, and 1,365 for the under-15s (table 23).

Road accidents are therefore and important factor in France's unenviable situation in terms of premature mortality. They represent the prime cause of death for the 15-24 age bracket: in 1996 they accounted for 39.6% of deaths among young men and 32.0% of deaths among young women in this age group. The considerable burden of road accidents among the young is also expressed by the fact that they not only represent 1.5% of general mortality but also 5.4% of premature mortality (death before the age of 65) and 9% of potential years of life lost.

The geographical context strongly affects the frequency of accidents involving bodily injury and the subsequent death toll. 70% of accidents take place in built-up areas and 30% in open country: on the other hand, of those killed, 34% are killed in built-up areas and 66% in open country. The gravity of accidents involving bodily injury, defined as the number of persons killed per hundred such accidents, is thus 4.5 times higher in open country. The lower mortality risk factor in highly built-up areas in large measure explains why the comparative mortality rate in the Île-de-France region is more than 10% lower than the French mean.

In order to take this whole array of causes into account, the French Interministerial Road Safety Surveillance Agency set out to study the types of French regions and "departments" (counties) as a function of numerous criteria known to be correlated with road hazards.

Table 23 **Relative risk of being killed or injured in a road accident as a function of age** (reference age group = 15-24-year-olds)

	killed	injured
0-14 years	0.13	0.20
15-24 years	1.00	1.00
25-44 years	0.59	0.52
45-64 years	0.42	0.31
65 years and over	0.58	0.23

Source: National Interministerial Road Safety Surveillance Agency.

The resulting document[9] is useful in allowing local participants to coherently judge their position relative to similar geographic areas in terms of accident data and hence better adapt their preventive measures.

Accidents in the workplace

Data concerning accidents in the workplace established by the management systems of the National Health Insurance Agency and the Agricultural Employees' Health Insurance Agency indicate that in 1996 a total of 703,000 occupational accidents occurred and involved an absence from work of at least 24 hours (in addition to the day of the accident itself), including 54,000 accidents which led to permanent disability and 870 deaths.

Variation in the number of stated occupational accidents and their repercussions

The 1996 results were the lowest ever recorded in terms of the number of accidents with time off work and the number of permanent disability pensions attributed (table 24). Only the number of deaths showed an increase relative to 1995; it should be pointed out that 40% of the deaths were due to road accidents, journeys between home and work being excluded.

The target set by the 1994 HCSP report was a reduction (regardless of its magnitude) in the number of accidents entailing time off work. This target has therefore been attained.

However, where this appreciation is concerned, it is important to take into account the difficulty of gauging the problems involved in declaration.

Given the year-to-year fluctuations in the job market, it is useful to express the number of occupational accidents with respect to the total number of hours worked (figure 10).

---

9. Observatoire national interministériel de sécurité routière (National Interministerial Road Safety Surveillance Agency), *"Typologie des régions et départements français pour l'aide à l'analyse en accidentologie"* (Typology of French regions and departments as an aid in analysing accidents), November 1995.

Indicators of health status

Table 24 **Morbidity and mortality due to occupational accidents**
(covers general and agricultural health insurance schemes)

	Accidents with time off work	Permanent disability	Death
1975	1,181,120	127,161	2,229
1980	1,030,877	109,527	1,571
1985	782,683	81,147	1,160
1990	808,415	73,844	1,287
1991	837,465	74,924	1,180
1992	798,143	68,738	1,112
1993	721,465	59,903	954
1994	713,065	61,608	909
1995	717,828	66,227	811
1996	702,865	53,837	869

Source: Cnamts and MSA.

Figure 10 **Frequency[a] of occupational accidents**

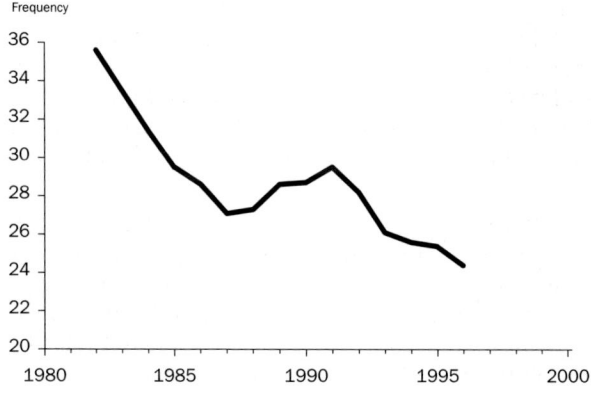

a. Frequency = number of accidents/number of hours worked × 1,000,000.
Source: Cnamts.

The calculated frequency showed an increase between 1987 and 1991 but has been continuously decreasing ever since.

The gravity index remained stationary between 1987 and 1991 and then started to decrease, though not as rapidly as during the period 1982-1987.

Figure 11 shows the variation in the mean gravity index of accidents – this is the ratio of all permanent disabilities officially recognized during the year to the number of hours worked.

Health in France / November 1998

Figure 11 **Gravity index[a] of permanent disabilities**

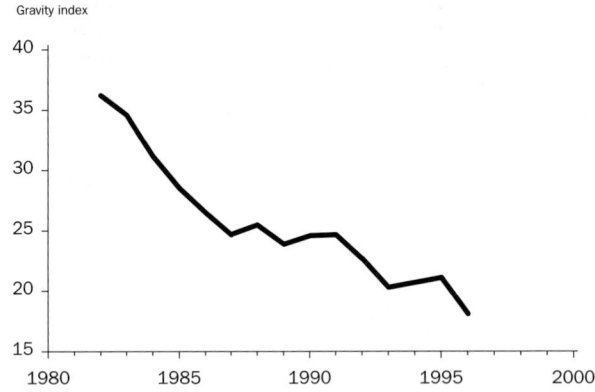

a. Gravity index = total of permanent disability rates/number of hours worked × 1,000,000.

Source: Cnamts.

SOURCES OF INFORMATION CONCERNING OCCUPATIONAL ACCIDENTS AND PROBLEMS IN DECLARATION

Available data concerning occupational accidents are derived from business data belonging to the general Social Security system and the Agricultural Employees' Health Insurance Agency. Hence they do not include occupational accidents that involve either shopkeepers, artisans and liberal professions, or employees covered by special schemes (French and overseas territorial civil service, SNCF (French national railways), etc.). They count the victims of occupational accidents recognised as being of a professional nature. Accordingly, the year corresponds to the date of recognition and differs from the year the accident occurred in an appreciable number of cases. Moreover, occupational accidents are only counted if they occasioned one day off from work in addition to the day on which the accident happened. It is estimated that for every accident counted in the statistics, 2.05 accidents actually happen. It is also highly probable that the employment situation and growing job insecurity work may lead to under-declaration of the actual number of accidents, whether or not they involve the loss of working days, particularly those which entail the fewest repercussions – this leads to an apparent rise in gravity indicators.

Indicators of health status

The number of working days lost due to temporary disability followed the same course as that of occupational accidents and decreased to 25.4 million in 1996 after having reached 28.5 million in 1991. However, considering the ratio of the total number of days lost to the number of accidents with time off work, it can be seen that the mean duration of time off work showed a regular increase, from 33.2 days in 1987 to 36.3 in 1991 and 38.6 in 1996. These results appear to confirm the idea of an under-declaration of accidents, particularly those which caused the shortest working day losses.

Factors affecting variations in frequency and gravity of occupational accidents

There is a wide variation in indicators, depending on the nature of the professional activity involved, from a frequency of 12.2 (chemical sector) to 58.9 (building and civil engineering), and from a gravity index of 7.9 (skins and leather) to 63.3 (building and civil engineering). The sectors most concerned in building and civil engineering are the wood industry and transport and handling. Metallurgy has the largest labour-force (2,050,000 employees), a frequency of 26.5 and a gravity index of 17.6.

In terms of professional qualifications, it can be seen that accidents happen primarily to manual workers, particularly unqualified manual workers. In fact, manual workers represented 36% of the labour force in 1995 but accounted for 78.5% of accidents with time off work. Accordingly, the global frequency of 25.4 for all personnel is based on a level of 55.4 for manual workers and 8.5 for the rest of the employees. The corresponding figures for unqualified manual workers are 11.3% of the labour force and 32.4% of accidents with time off work. The frequency among manual workers then reaches 46.6 for those who are qualified and 72.8 for those who are unqualified.

In 1995, foreign employees represented 6.6% of the labour force but 11.3% of accidents with time off work and 16.1% of accidents with permanent disability (table 25).

However, given that foreign workers are very unevenly distributed in the various sectors of activity, it might be thought that these results merely reflect the fact that very large numbers work in the most exposed sectors. In actual fact, when the results for the metallurgy and building sectors are examined, it is seen that the risk among foreign workers is very much higher than that of French workers engaged in the same professional sector in terms of both gravity and frequency. This might be attributable to the fact that those concerned are generally poorly qualified and, in addition, may have difficulties in adapting.

Age is also an important factor affecting variations in occupational accidents. The frequency of accidents with time off work is markedly higher in those over 30. On the other hand, gravity as measured by the mean duration of temporary disability or the mean rate of permanent disability shows a regular increase with age (table 26).

Table 25 **Percentage of foreign employees[a] in the labour force and involved in accidents in 1995**

	Labour force[b]	Accidents with time off work	Accidents with permanent disability	Days lost due to temporary disability	Rate of permanent disability
All activities	6.6	11.3	16.1	15.2	16.1
Metallurgy	5.7	9.8	13.1	11.9	12.5
Civil engineering and building	16.9	19.9	29.1	26.8	29.1

a. Including the European Union.
b. Source: INSEE employment survey.
Source: Cnamts.

Table 26 **Gravity indicators for occupational accidents as a function of age in 1995**

	Mean duration of temporary disability (days)	Mean rate of permanent disability (%)
20-24 years	25.3	8.5
25-29 years	30.3	8.5
30-34 years	36.2	8.9
35-39 years	41.7	8.9
40-49 years	49.2	9.6
50-59 years	59.6	10.1

Source: Cnamts.

Cancer

Cancer is the second cause of mortality in France after cardiovascular disease, and the first cause of premature mortality (before the age of 65). The value of having data on the incidence of cancer readily available no longer needs to be demonstrated. For the first time, a study of cancer registers (see box) has made it possible to estimate the incidence of the most common cancers over time for the entire population. The estimates were made for the period 1990-1995 and the changes observed during this period do not completely coincide in terms of mortality with the changes previously described for the period 1991-1996.

Cancer-related mortality and the incidence of cancer in France in 1995

In France, cancer was responsible for **142,635 deaths**, including 61% of deaths among men, **in 1995**. In descending order of frequency, cancer affected the lungs (24,000 deaths), colorectum (16,000 deaths), the upper airways and digestive tract (12,000 deaths), blood and blood-forming tissues (11,000 deaths), and breast (11,000 deaths). Malignant cancer was the first cause of mortality among men (29% of all deaths) and the second among women, after cardiovascular disease (23% of all deaths) with, respectively, a comparative rate (standardised relative to the French population in 1990) of 374 per 100,000 men and 165 per 100,000 women. Above all, it accounted for 26% of premature mortality before the age of 65 in men and 29% in women. It is estimated that a total of **239,800 new cases** of cancer were discovered in 1995, including 56% among men. The most frequent location was in the breast (34,000 cases), followed by the colon and rectum (33,000 cases), the prostate (26,000 cases) then, in equal measure, the lung and upper airways and digestive tract (22,000 cases).

For 1995, the estimated comparative incidence was 552 per 100,000 men and 326 per 100,000 women. The ratio of incidence to mortality can hence be evaluated at 1.5 among males and 2 for females, which indicates that on the whole women have a better chance of surviving cancer than men. In those under 65, the incidence is estimated to be 210 per 100,000 men (38% of the total incidence) and 173 per 100,000 women (53% of the total incidence).

In men, four locations are each responsible for over 15,000 new cases per year: cancer of the prostate heads the list, followed by two locations with a poor prognosis directly related to excessive alcohol consumption and smoking, *i.e.* cancer of the upper airways and digestive tract, and lung cancer. Colorectal cancer occupies fourth place. The ranking differs in terms of mortality and lung cancer comes first by a wide margin as the cause of over 20,000 deaths. It is followed by cancer of the UADT, responsible for more than 10,000 deaths, then prostate and colorectal cancers. The number of deaths due to lung cancer is certainly overestimated since a certain number of cases probably involve a lung metastasis and not a primary lung cancer. This would explain the excess of deaths relative to the incidence of lung cancer.

In women, breast cancer is by far the most frequent form of cancer with more than 33,000 new cases in 1995, followed by colorectal cancer, then haematological cancer and gynaecological cancer with a relatively good prognosis. In terms of mortality, the same first three locations are found as before, with lung cancer in fourth position. As in men, the number of deaths attributed to lung cancer is certainly overestimated, as is the incidence of lung cancer, a certain number of cases involving a lung metastasis and not a primary lung cancer.

Part two Changes in health status

ESTIMATION OF CANCER INCIDENCE IN FRANCE*

It is important to dispose of data concerning morbidity due to cancer for the purposes of deciding on, and monitoring, public health measures. The corresponding mortality rates are inadequate for this, given the modifications introduced by altered conditions of diagnosis, variable post-treatment survival and especially recovery.

The incidence of cancer in France is estimated by taking the incidence actually observed in geographic areas covered by a cancer register and extrapolating the regional data using mortality and demographic data available for the whole country.

Assuming a certain hypothetical stability, this conventionally used method of modelling the ratio of incidence to mortality makes it possible to extrapolate.

The estimates given in the present report concern the period 1990-1995 and the data relating to incidence were derived from eleven general and specialised registers covering nine departments: Bas-Rhin, Calvados, Côte-d'Or, Doubs, Haut-Rhin, Hérault, Isère, Somme, and Tarn.

* Menegoz F., et al., Cancer incidence and mortality in France in 1975-1995, Eur J Cancer Prev 1997; 6: 442-466.

Variation in mortality and the incidence of cancer between 1990 and 1995

Cancer-related **mortality in men** has been increasing steadily since 1950 and rose by + 3% between 1990 and 1995, while premature mortality (under 65) decreased by − 9%. The fall in premature mortality was basically due to major decreases in premature mortality caused by cancer of the (i) UADT (− 27%) following a drop in alcohol consumption, and (ii) prostate gland (− 24%), and also to more modest decreases in colorectal cancer (− 5%) and lung cancer (− 1.4%). There has also been a more moderate increase in deaths due to lung cancer, thanks to a reduction in smoking, and a decrease in carcinoma of the stomach due to improved eating habits. Since 1975, there has been a regular increase in the **estimated incidence** of cancer (initial data estimates were based on data from cancer registers): the comparative incidence increased by more than 21% between 1975 and 1995 but was relatively stable between 1990 and 1995.

Cancer-related mortality among women has gradually slowed down since 1975 (− 9% in 20 years), but showed a moderate increase of about + 4% between 1990 and 1995, whereas a decrease in premature mortality (under 65) of more than − 3% was noted during the same period. In part, the latter reduction was due to a decrease in premature mortality due to colorectal cancer (− 13%) and cancer of the cervix (− 8%). The general increase in the mortality rate can be explained by the increase in deaths due to lung cancer (related to smoking) and cancer of the UADT, and also by a slight rise in breast cancer. **The estimated incidence of cancer in women** has been steadily increasing since

Indicators of health status

1975: the standardised incidence has risen by more than 16% in 20 years. Between 1990 and 1995, as in men, there was a more modest increase in incidence than mortality, less than + 0.5% per year.

In its 1994 report, the High Committee on Public Health set targets for the reduction in mortality rates due to cancer in six different locations, each being selected for the weight of its contribution to total mortality and/or the recognized possibility of prevention through early screening. The following paragraphs indicate the changes that have been observed in the incidence and mortality associated with the various cancers.

Lung cancer[10]

In 1995, lung cancer was responsible for almost 24,000 deaths, including 85% in men, thereby making it the prime location for cancer. The estimated number of new cases is close on 22,000, including 86% among males, putting lung cancer in fourth place in terms of incidence.

In 1995, the comparative mortality rates for lung cancer were 83 per 100,000 men and 11 per 100,000 women, and lung cancer accounted for 28% of cancer-related premature mortality in men and 8% in women. In 1990, it was responsible for respectively 26% and 6% of premature mortality due to cancer. The comparative estimated incidence in 1995 was 72 per 100,000 men and 10 per 100,000 women, giving a *sex ratio* of 7.2. The onset of lung cancer rarely occurs in those under 45. Its cumulative incidence between 0 and 64 years is estimated at 36 per 100,000 men and 5 per 100,000 women, *i.e.* more than half the total incidence.

Although there was an overall + 5% increase in the mortality rate due to lung cancer in men between 1990 and 1995, the premature mortality rate decreased by – 1%. The estimated incidence decreased by – 3% between 1990 and 1995. Over the same period, overall mortality, premature mortality and the estimated incidence of lung cancer in women all underwent an increase of about + 20%. The increase in incidence was particularly marked among young women (+ 43% in women 25-44 years old).

If the trend observed between 1990 and 1995 continues, the targeted decrease of – 15% in mortality due to lung cancer will obviously be unattainable by the year 2010 (figure 12).

---

10. Code 162 in the "Classification internationale des maladies" (CIM) (International Classification of Diseases), 9th revision.

Figure 12 **Mortality due to lung cancer (all ages)**
(comparative rates smoothed over 3-year periods)

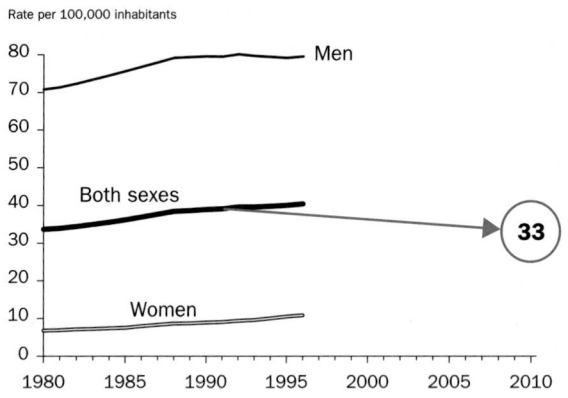

Source: Inserm SC8.

A steep increase in cases among women is to be feared, similar to that which occurred in the United States, unless suitable prevention programmes aimed at young women are stepped up: the French comparative mortality rate due to lung cancer is currently similar to the rate noted in the United States in the middle of the 1960s. The latter has tripled in 15 years and, in 1990, exceeded the mortality rate due to breast cancer, placing it first among cancer-related deaths in women.

Cancer of the upper airways and digestive tract[11] (UADT)

In 1995, cancer of the UADT was responsible for more than 12,000 deaths, including 87% in men, thereby putting it in third place in terms of cancer-related mortality, after lung cancer and colorectal cancer. Cancer of the lips, mouth and pharynx were the most common, accounting for 43% of deaths due to cancer of the UADT, followed by cancer of the œsophagus (38%) and larynx (19%). The estimated number of new cases was almost 22,000, including 88% in men, so that these locations came in fifth position in terms of incidence. Incident cases and deaths differed in their breakdown: cancer of the lips, mouth and pharynx represented 58% of the cases, followed by an equal number of cases of cancer of the œsophagus and larynx. In terms of both incidence and mortality, there was a marked predominance in women of cancer of the lips, mouth and pharynx, at the expense of cancer of the larynx. Two thirds of cases of cancer of the UADT were said to be attributable to smoking, and 8 cancers in 10 to alcohol.

---

11. Included under the heading of the term "cancers of the UADT (upper airways and digestive tract)" are cancers of the lips, buccal cavity, pharynx, œsophagus and larynx. Codes 140-149, 150-161 of the CIM 9th revision.

The comparative mortality rates due to cancer of the UADT in 1995 were 42 per 100,000 men and 5 per 100,000 women. This type of cancer accounted for 19% of cancer-related premature mortality in men and 4% in women. In 1990, it was responsible for respectively 22% and 4% of the premature mortality due to cancer. In 1995, the comparative incidence was 72 per 100,000 men and 8 per 100,000 women, giving a *sex ratio* of 9. This type of cancer is relatively rare in those under 45. The cumulative incidence between 0 and 64 years was estimated at 41 per 100,000 men and 4 per 100,000 women, *i.e.* 57 and 58% of the total incidence respectively.

While the mortality rate due to cancer of the UADT showed an overall decrease of – 17% in men between 1990 and 1995, the decrease in the premature mortality rate was greater (– 27%). Over the same period, the incidence showed a similar downward trend estimated at – 15%. A very much smaller overall decrease in mortality was noted in women than in men (about – 2%) between 1990 and 1995, without any reduction in premature mortality and above all an augmentation in the estimated incidence of + 8%.

If the trend in mortality observed between 1990 and 1995 continues, it can be predicted that the target of reducing mortality due to cancer of the UADT by – 30% by the year 2010 could be achieved (figure 13). However, the changes will not occur in parallel in men and women, though the differences between the two sexes are narrowing as patterns in alcohol- and smoking-related risk factors change in France, *i.e.* a generalised decline in alcohol consumption and stable smoking level due to a decrease

Figure 13 **Mortality due to cancer of the upper airways and digestive tract (all ages)**
(comparative rates smoothed over 3-year periods)

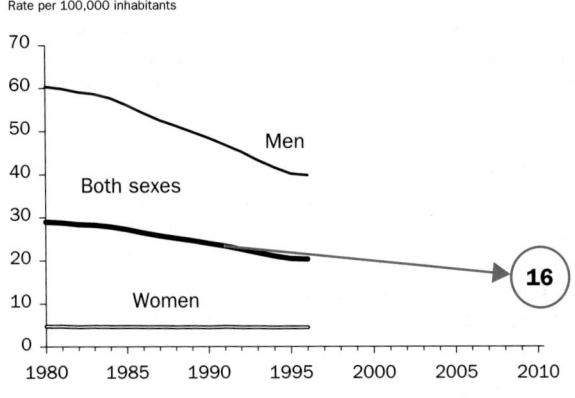

Source: *Inserm SC8.*

Part two   Changes in health status

among men and an increase among women. In practice, preventing smoking might be the most effective means of limiting the rise in the number of cancers of the UADT among women.

Breast cancer[12] In 1995, breast cancer was responsible for almost 11,000 deaths, putting it in fifth place in terms of mortality due to cancer. The estimated number of new cases is close to 34,000, making breast cancer the most common cancer among women.

The comparative mortality rate due to breast cancer in women in 1995 was 33 per 100,000. This type of cancer accounted for 30% of cancer-related premature mortality in women in 1995, and 28% in 1990. The comparative estimated incidence was 108 per 100,000 in 1995, giving an incidence/mortality ratio of 3.3. The estimated cumulative incidence between 0 and 64 years was calculated to be 73 per 100,000, *i.e.* 68% of the total incidence.

Although the mortality rate due to breast cancer showed a slight overall increase between 1990 and 1995 (+ 3%), the premature mortality rate remained practically stable (+ 1%). This increase in premature mortality affected young women (+ 4% among those 25-44 years old) and particularly elderly women over 74 (+ 8%). In the other age brackets, the mortality rate showed instead a tendency to decrease slightly. During the same period, the estimated incidence increased by + 16%, *i.e.* an annual variation of about 3%. Such tendencies must be seen in the light of earlier diagnosis, notably in the context of routine screening programmes for breast cancer (see chapter 6), and an improvement in treatment efficacy and patient quality of life.

If the trend noted between 1990 and 1995 continues, the targeted decrease of − 30% in mortality due to breast cancer among women aged 50-70 by the year 2010 might not be achieved (figure 14). However, a positive start to a decrease in mortality has been noted for this age group.

Cervical cancer[13] In 1995, cervical cancer was responsible for about 1,600 deaths and the estimated number of new cases was almost 3,300.

The comparative mortality rate due to cervical cancer in 1995 was 4.8 per 100,000, and cervical cancer had practically the same weight in terms of cancer-related premature mortality as in 1990. The comparative estimated incidence in 1995 was 10.5 per 100,000. The cumulative incidence between 0 and 64 years was estimated at 7.4 per 100,000, *i.e.* 77% of the total incidence.

Between 1990 and 1995, there was an overall decrease of − 4% in the mortality rate due to cervical cancer. The decline in mortality

---
12. Codes 174-175 of the CIM 9th revision.
13. Code 180 of the CIM 9th revision after correction for cases of uterine cancer with unspecified site.

Figure 14 **Mortality due to breast cancer (50-69 years)**
(comparative rates smoothed over 3-year periods)

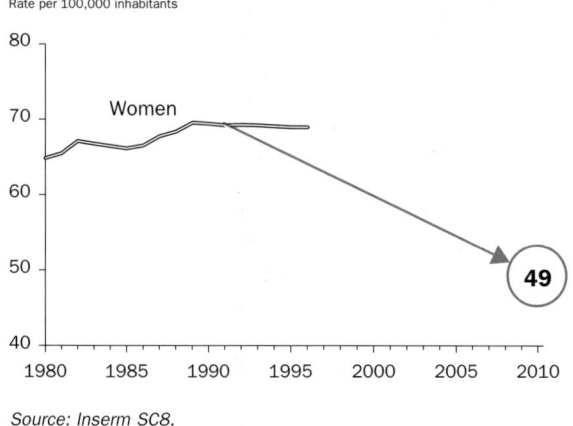

Source: Inserm SC8.

appears to have been more marked among women over 44. The decrease in the estimated incidence during the same period was high, – 13%, *i.e.* an annual variation of about – 3%. The increased incidence recently observed among young women (under 35) in some Northern European countries has not been reported in France.

If the trend noted between 1990 and 1995 continues in terms of **all** deaths due to uterine cancer, it can be predicted that the expected 30% decrease is attainable by the year 2010 (figure 15).

Figure 15 **Mortality due to uterine cancer (all ages)**
(comparative rates smoothed over 3-year periods)

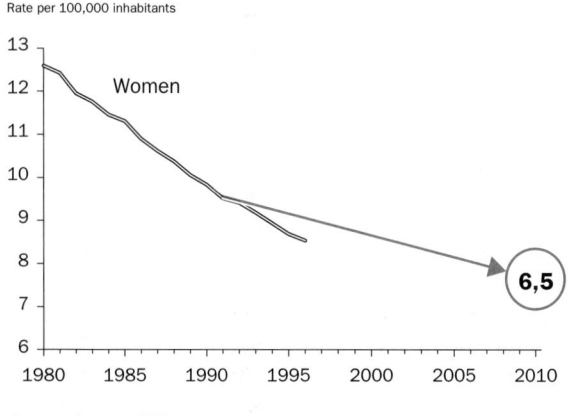

Source: Inserm SC8.

Part two   Changes in health status

Colorectal cancer[14]

In 1995, colorectal cancer was responsible for more than 16,000 deaths, including 52% in men. It accounted for 7% of cancer-related premature mortality among men and 8% among women. The number of new cases was estimated at over 33,000, including 54% in men. In terms of both mortality and incidence, the colorectum is the second most frequent location for cancer.

In 1995, the comparative mortality rates for colorectal cancer were 38 per 100,000 men and 22 per 100,000 women. Colorectal cancer accounted for 19% of cancer-related premature mortality in men and 4% in women. The comparative incidence in 1995 was 75 per 100,000 men and 46 per 100,000 women, giving a *sex ratio* of 1.6. Colorectal cancer rarely occurs in those under 45 but its onset increases exponentially with age. Between 0 and 64 years, its cumulative incidence is estimated to be 25 per 100,000 men and 16 per 100,000 women, *i.e.* respectively 33% and 34% of the total incidence.

Figure 16   **Mortality due to colorectal cancer (all ages)**
(comparative rates smoothed over 3-year periods)

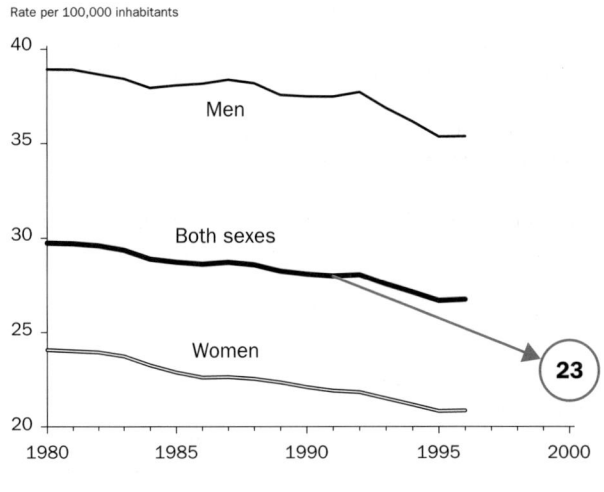

Source: Inserm SC8.

In men, while the mortality rate due to colorectal cancer showed an overall increase of + 3% between 1990 and 1995, the premature mortality rate declined by – 5% (– 14% among those aged 25-44, – 4% among those aged 45-64). The estimated incidence increased by 12% between 1990 and 1995. During the same period, an overall decrease in mortality of about 4% was noted in

---

14. Codes 153-154 of the CIM 9th revision.

women, accompanied by a 13% decrease in premature mortality while, as in men, there was an increase of about 13% in the estimated incidence, primarily due to an augmentation in cancer of the right colon. These divergent changes in incidence and mortality were attributed to much earlier diagnosis and advances in treatment, especially for carcinoma of the colon.

If the trend in mortality noted between 1990 and 1995 continues, the target of a 10% decrease is unlikely to be achieved by the year 2000, except perhaps among young men (figure 16). In women, in spite of a marked decrease in premature mortality, the target will be difficult to attain. In terms of prevention, current efforts must be continued and stepped up.

Melanoma[15]

In 1995, melanoma was responsible for more than 1,100 deaths, including 50% in men, and the estimated number of new cases was more than 4,200, including 41% in men. The most common anatomical sites of melanoma were the lower limbs in women and the trunk in men.

The comparative mortality rates due to melanoma in 1995 were 2.3 per 100,000 men and 1.7 per 100,000 women. In 1995, melanoma accounted for 1% of cancer-related premature mortality in men and 1.7% in women. In 1990, it was responsible for respectively 0.8% and 1.6% of premature mortality due to cancer. The comparative incidence in 1995 was 6.4 per 100,000 men and 8 per 100,000 women, giving a *sex ratio* of 0.8. The cumulative incidence between 0 and 64 years was estimated at 4.4 per 100,000 men and 5.7 per 100,000 women, *i.e.* respectively 68% and 69% of the total incidence. These data indicate improved survival in women, which must be seen in parallel with their greater vigilance with respect to lesions arising on more accessible sites (lower limbs) which, moreover, makes the medical monitoring of asymptomatic nævi easier.

There was an overall 9% increase in the mortality rate due to melanoma among men between 1990 and 1995, accompanied by a slightly higher increase in the premature mortality rate of 10% (the increase was even more pronounced among 25-44-year-olds: + 17%). In women, during the same period, an overall increase of about 6% was noted in the mortality rate, without any variation in premature mortality. The largest increase occurred in the 65-74 age group (+ 25%). The estimated incidence increased by 7% in men and 4% in women between 1990 and 1995.

If the trend observed between 1990 and 1995 continues, it will be difficult to attain the target of stabilising mortality due to melanoma by the year 2000 (figure 17). Primary prevention must

---

15. Code 172 of the CIM 9th revision.

Part two Changes in health status

be maintained and, to increase effectiveness, secondary prevention could be aimed at each individual sex.

Figure 17 **Mortality due to melanoma (all ages)**
(comparative rates smoothed over 3-year periods)

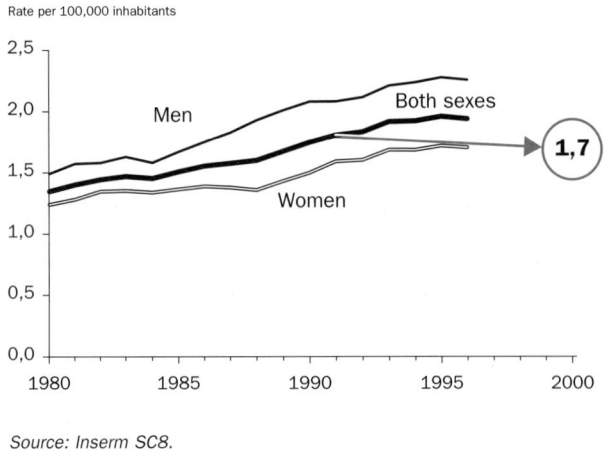

Source: Inserm SC8.

Regional disparities in cancer-related mortality in 1995

In 1995, **inter-regional disparities in mortality** due to cancer were greater among men than women:
– in men, comparative mortality rates ranged respectively from – 16% lower mortality in the Midi-Pyrénées region to + 26% excess mortality in the Nord-Pas-de-Calais region. Regions with excess general cancer-related mortality were the Champagne-Ardenne region and all those regions which had excess premature mortality rates 10% higher than the national mean;
– in women, variations in the comparative rates were more modest than in men (– 12% to + 14%). As in men, the Nord-Pas-de-Calais region was particularly affected by cancer-related deaths, and the excess premature mortality among women was + 19%.

Between 1990 and 1995, regional disparities showed the following variations:
– in men, three out of five regions with excess mortality due to cancer 10% higher than the national mean between 1990 and 1995 had a rate of increase higher than the French mean increase (+ 3%): the regions concerned were Picardy (+ 8%), and Nord-Pas-de-Calais and Brittany (+ 6%). However, on a positive note, a greater decrease (about – 12%) than the French mean decrease (– 9%) has been observed in terms of premature mortality in the Nord-Pas-de-Calais and Brittany regions. Special attention must be paid to Poitou-Charentes which is the only region with a mortality rate more than 10% below the national mean and saw a 5%

Indicators of health status

increase in its premature mortality rate due to cancer between 1990 and 1995;

— in women, unlike the situation observed in men, there were wide regional variations in overall mortality rates due to cancer between 1990 and 1995, ranging from − 8% in the Limousin to + 10% in the Pays-de-la-Loire. Similarly, the premature mortality rates varied from − 21% in the Limousin to − 13% in Corsica. There was a considerable increase in premature mortality between 1990 and 1995 in a certain number of regions that had a lower mortality rate relative to the national mean, notably the Auvergne and Poitou-Charentes. Conversely, some regions with excess cancer-related mortality rates, such Picardy and Alsace, saw a decrease in their premature mortality due to cancer between 1990 and 1995.

European comparisons of mortality and the incidence of cancer in 1990

In men, the most marked differences between European countries in 1990 were in terms of the incidence of cancer rather than cancer-related mortality. Cancer rates were particularly high in France and comparable to those in the Netherlands (figure 18).

In women, France occupied a position among those countries with average rates, similar to those noted in southern European countries. Without having any more recent data, it is impossible to discuss the changes in these countries' rates between 1990 and 1995 (figure 18).

Figure 18 **Comparative incidence and mortality due to cancers (except skin cancer) in various countries of the European Union in 1990**

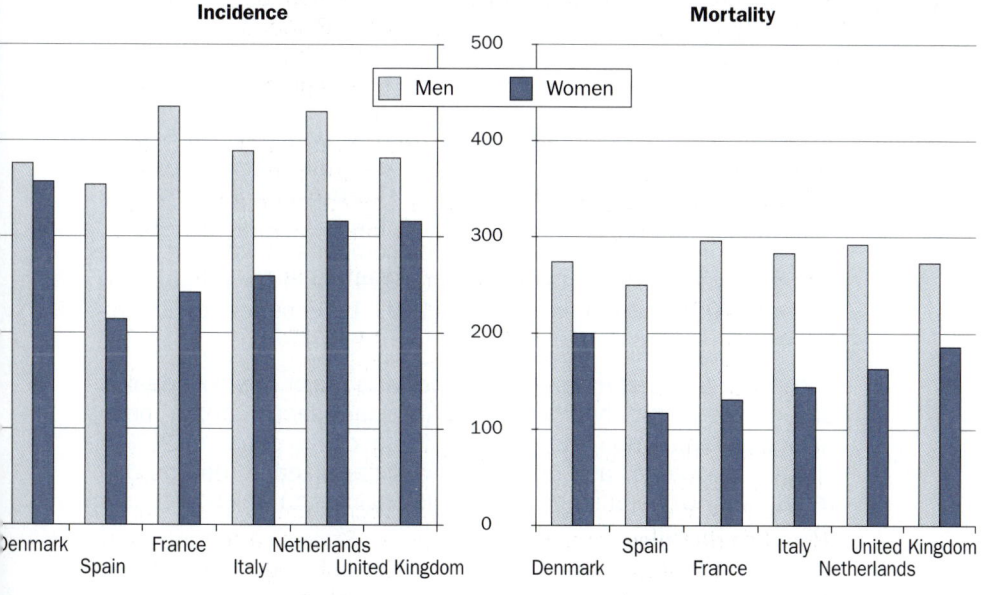

Cardiovascular disease

Cardiovascular diseases (or diseases of the circulatory system) are the prime cause of mortality in France, and they are also the diseases most frequently declared by the population, after oral and dental conditions and ophthalmological problems. They constitute the most common reason for consulting a doctor in private practice (see the chapter *Indicators of health status, "Morbidity"*).

The onset of cardiovascular conditions depends, to a great extent, on age and, for some of them, on a combination of several risk factors – constitutional susceptibility, individual behaviour patterns, and environmental conditions – which affect the circulatory system throughout life before any clinical signs become apparent.

It is generally accepted that a large number of cardiovascular conditions, especially in those under 75, could be avoided by adopting measures that combine screening and appropriate treatment for hyperlipidaemia, hypertension and diabetes, and also anti-smoking campaigns.

In its 1994 General Report on *Health in France*, the High Committee on Public Health set itself the target of reducing mortality due to cardiovascular diseases by 20% among persons under 75 years of age before the year 2000.

Changes in cardiovascular mortality

Cardiovascular causes as a whole were responsible for 173,128 deaths in France in 1996, including 44,141 among those under 75.

Since 1991, mortality rates have shown a marked decrease of – 10% for all ages combined, and a greater decrease among women (– 12%) than among men (– 8%). The decrease was slightly greater among the under 75s (– 12%), with rates lowered by 14% among women and 11% among men. However, these variations in the under-75s mark a slowdown in the fall of deaths due to diseases of the circulatory system by comparison with the previous period. The HCSP target set in 1994 could be achieved by the year 2000 if the present trend (1991-1996 period) continues (figure 19).

The circulation disorders responsible for a major share of deaths are (i) ischaemic heart disease (sudden death, death post-myocardial infarction, etc.) which is the declared cause of 27% of circulatory deaths, and (ii) cerebrovascular disease (deaths due to stroke of ischaemic, haemorrhagic origin, etc.) which accounts for 25% of deaths.

Figure 19 **Mortality due to cardiovascular disease in under-75s**
(comparative rates smoothed over 3-year periods)

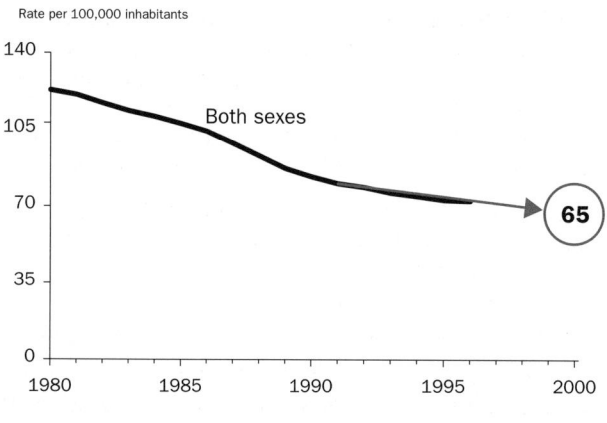

Source: Inserm SC8.

Ischaemic heart disease

In 1996, 47,267 deaths were due to ischaemic heart disease, including 16,078 among persons under 75. In common with all causes of death, there has been an appreciable drop in the mortality rates due to ischaemic heart disease since 1991, – 11% for all ages combined and – 15% for those under 75, with women having the greater advantage (respectively – 14% and – 17%). Nevertheless, this notable decrease is very much below the decrease which characterized the preceding period, especially the years 1985-1990 (figure 20).

Figure 20 **Mortality due to ischaemic heart disease**
(under 75s, comparative rates smoothed over 3-year periods)

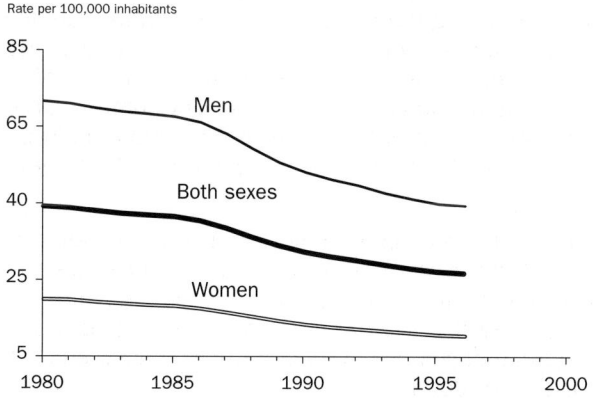

Source: Inserm SC8.

Part two Changes in health status

An analysis of the comparative rates reveals considerable regional inequalities, with excess mortality among both males and females affecting all of Brittany, and Northern and Eastern France. In these regions, the mortality rates due to ischaemic heart disease are more than 10% higher than the national mean (figure 21).

Monica-France registers give indications concerning mortality, morbidity, lethality and requests for medical care for myocardial infarction in France over the period 1985-1993 (see box on opposite page). At the present time, such data can only be obtained from disease registers: however, they only cover three geographic regions of limited size (1,000,000 inhabitants each).

Figure 21 **Ischaemic heart disease as a function of the region**
(1992-1994, comparative mortality rates)

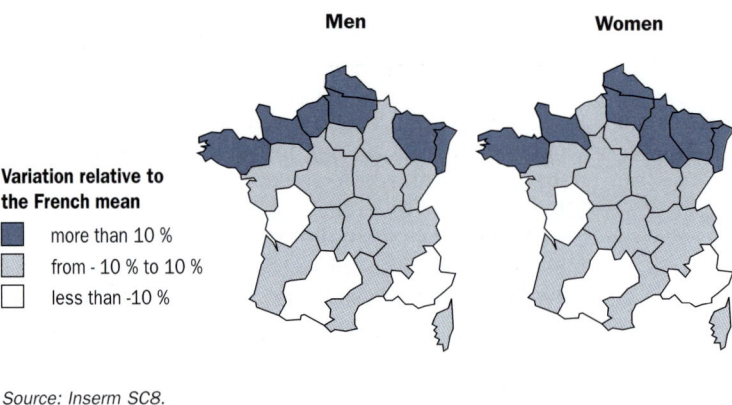

Variation relative to the French mean
- more than 10 %
- from -10 % to 10 %
- less than -10 %

Source: Inserm SC8.

REGISTERS OF MYOCARDIAL INFARCTION MONICA-FRANCE NETWORK

France took part in the WHO Monica project which monitors the longitudinal trends in the incidence of myocardial infarction and mortality due to coronary heart disease and their determinants over a 10-year period in specified geographic areas. Subjects aged under 65 were registered in accordance with a standardised protocol that included validation procedures. In France, the urban community of Lille and the Bas-Rhin and Haute-Garonne regions were involved and the full results are available for the three centres covering the period 1985-1993. A simplified presentation of the results was published in a booklet by the "Fédération française de cardiologie" (French Cardiology Federation) ("l'infarctus du myocarde en France", 1996 (Myocardial infarction in France, 1996)).

On the whole, the mortality rate due to ischaemic heart disease in the three regions was slightly higher than that given for the same regions by national death statistics, as is to be expected (table 27).

Table 27 **Age-adjusted mortality due to ischaemic heart disease in all three Monica regions, data from registers and data from national statistics, as a function of sex**
(35-64 years, annual rates per 100,000)

	1985	1989	1993
Men			
Monica regions	93.3	78.4	67.2
French regional statistics	98.7	75.6	60.0
France as a whole	79.8	62.8	54.6
Women			
Monica regions	19.2	13.9	13.8
French regional statistics	16.6	13.1	11.2
France as a whole	13.6	11.1	9.1

Source: Monica-France, SC 8 Inserm.

When the three regions are considered as a single group, the coronary mortality rate is systematically found to be higher than that for France as a whole. There was a spectacular drop in coronary mortality between 1985 and 1993 (about 30%), irrespective of sex. There are probably differences in the changes that take place in each region – for example, this decrease in the mortality rate was not found in Lille.

The incidence of myocardial infarction in both sexes fell during the period 1985-1993, though to a far lesser extent (between 8 and 10%) than the mortality rate (table 28).

It fell for both hospitalised and non hospitalised cases, and the proportion of non hospitalised cases (in practice, subjects who died before reaching hospital) showed a slight decrease (from 15.4% in 1985 to 13.7% in 1993).

Hence, the considerable improvement in coronary mortality during this period implies that, in addition, the lethality of myocardial infarction in hospitalised patients had greatly diminished; this is

Table 28 **Age-adjusted incidence of myocardial infarction in all three Monica regions, as a function of whether patient hospitalisation was possible or not**
(35-64 years, annual rate per 100,000)

	1985	1989	1993
Men			
Hospitalised	163.6	146.5	153.5
Not hospitalised	29.0	29.0	24.5
Women			
Hospitalised	28.5	25.7	26.7
Not hospitalised	6.1	5.7	4.2

Source: Monica-France.

shown in table 29, with lethality dropping from 23% to 18% between the two extreme periods. It is remarkable that, at the same time, there was a slight reduction in the time to hospitalisation and that, above all, there were considerable changes in hospital management procedures for the disease. With increasing frequency, arterial patency was restored by more aggressive intervention, and the administration of drugs with proven efficacy such as β-blockers and aspirin was initiated. However, these average changes conceal considerable inter-regional differences. For example, no improvement in hospital lethality was observed in Lille, and much slower progress was made in terms of management in Strasbourg than in other regions.

Table 29 **Characteristics of hospital management of myocardial infarction in the three Monica regions, after adjustment for age and sex (as a percentage)**

	1985-1987	1989-1990	1993
Died in hospital[a]	23.4	18.5	17.8
Time to hospitalisation less than 6 h	b	54.5	56.5
Coronary arteriogram	45.1	67.4	74.7
Angioplasty	6.5	24.3	37.3
Fibrinolytic therapy	19.8	31.2	34.2
β-blockers	31.9	54.0	68.7
Aspirin	b	68.4	79.8

a. Death occurred within 28 days after the onset of symptoms.
b. Data unavailable.
Source: Monica-France.

More recent data are not yet available. Nevertheless, it seems feasible to assume that these trends have continued and probably equally account for the persistent drop in cardiovascular mortality observed up until 1996. It would be more difficult to make extrapolations for subsequent periods.

Cerebrovascular disease

43,455 deaths were due to cerebrovascular disease in 1996, all ages combined, including 9,856 among those under 75.

It is in this domain that the most striking decreases were recorded: – 18% for all ages combined, essentially because of two age groups, 45-65-year-olds (– 21%) and over-74s (– 19%).

In those under 75, mortality rates dropped by a total of 15% (17% among women and 14% among men). As with other cardiovascular conditions, the reductions noted in terms of cerebrovascular disease were not as marked as in earlier periods (figure 22).

Indicators of health status

Figure 22 **Mortality due to cerebrovascular disease**
(under 75s, comparative rates smoothed over 3-year periods)

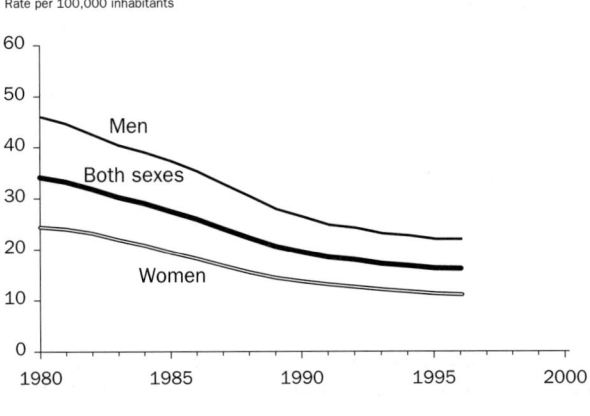

Source: Inserm SC8.

A regional analysis also revealed differences, though differences exceeding 10% concerned a more limited number of regions. These were always in northern France, apart from two exceptions: the Limousin and Corsica, where the mortality rates were higher than the national mean (figure 23).

Figure 23 **Cerebrovascular disease as a function of the region**
(1992-1994, comparative mortality rates

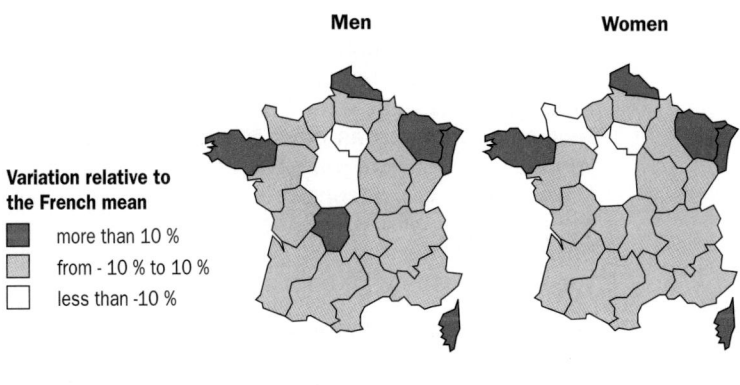

Source: Inserm SC8.

Changes in stated cardiovascular morbidity

There are few sources of data in France which can serve as the basis for determining the prevalence of cardiovascular diseases and especially the variations that they undergo. The only available national surveys are based on statements by individuals or the

Health in France / November 1998

reasons for medical consultations and hence do not reflect actual morbidity (see the chapter *Indicators of health status, "Morbidity"*).

Cardiovascular diseases are among those conditions most frequently declared by individuals. In terms of prevalence, they affected 28% of men and 37% of women in the period 1992-1995. With respect to the period 1988-1991, this amounts to a progression of + 25% for men and 11% for women (table 30).

Table 30 **Variation in the declared prevalence of cardiovascular diseases as a function of the nature of the disease, 1988-1991 to 1992-1995** (all ages included, comparison rates for 100 persons)

	Men		Women	
	1992-1996	Variation 92-95/88-91	1992-1996	Variation 92-95/88-91
Hypertension	10.5	25%*	11.1	1%
Ischaemic heart disease	3.0	– 4%	2.1	– 3%
Other heart diseases	3.4	7%	2.9	– 21%*
Cerebrovascular diseases	1.9	> 100%*	2.4	> 100%*
including stroke	0.6	13%	0.4	– 9%
Diseases of arteries and arterioles	2.6	28%	1.2	6%
Venous and lymphatic diseases	6.7	31%*	17.5	17%*
All cardiovascular diseases	**28.0**	**25%***	**37.16**	**11%***

Reading: in 1992-1995, 10.5% of men stated that they had hypertension, *i.e.* a 25% increase relative to 1988-1991. The variations marked with an asterisk(*) indicate a 95% significant difference in the raw data between the two four-year periods.
Source: CREDES, ESPS survey 1988-1991/1992-1995.

The most frequent conditions do not correspond to the causes of mortality: in fact, venous disease and hypertension top the declarations made by both men and women. However, although hypertension is declared as often by men as by women (about 10%), venous disorders are more than twice as frequent among women (18% *versus* 7%). Among men, there was a marked increase in the frequency with which these two disorders were declared in between the two periods. Among women, only declarations of venous diseases showed a significant increase.

The progression noted in cerebrovascular disease, including its declaration, was multiplied by 2.9 in men and 4.2 in women, in keeping with the observed reduction in mortality due to this cause. In fact, it is basically accounted for by an increase in declarations of "cerebrovascular insufficiency", related to the instigation of numerous "vasculoprotective" treatments which improve capillary function. Declarations of strokes as strictly defined appear to have been stable between the two periods but were too few in number in our surveys for any trend to be noted.

Indicators of health status

The prevalence of ischaemic heart disease is stable and the slight decrease observed in both men and women is not significant. However, the decrease is in line with the fall in mortality and might indicate an actual decrease in the incidence of ischaemic heart disease.

Changes in the frequency of cardiovascular reasons for consulting a doctor in private practice

Cardiovascular disease is very often the reason why a patient consults a doctor (table 31).

In 1996, cardiovascular disease was mentioned 26 and 33 times respectively per 100 sessions given by (i) any type of specialist or (ii) a general practitioner. The most frequent was hypertension, mentioned 13 times per 100 GP sessions, followed by venous and lymphatic disorders, 7.6; ischaemic heart disease, 3.7; and "other heart diseases", 3.8 times per 100.

Between 1992 and 1996, the variations observed were structurally minimal among both GPs and specialists. Significant but small drops were noted among GPs in terms of the number of consultations for hypertension and cerebrovascular disorders. In contrast, there was an increase in the relative frequency of venous and lymphatic disorders. It should also be noted that, as a result of the increased total number of sessions per year, + 12,6%, there was a parallel rise in the number of sessions involving at least one cardiovascular disease (from 61.3 to 66.4 million per year).

Table 31 **Consultation of a doctor in private practice for a cardiovascular disease**

(number of diagnoses per 100 sessions)

	GPs		Specialists		Total	
	1996	Variation 1992-1996	1996	Variation 1992-1996	1996	Variation 1992-1996
Hypertension	13.4	– 3%*	2.0	– 4%	10.0	– 4%
Ischaemic heart disease	3.7	– 5%	1.7	15%	3.1	– 2%
Other heart diseases	3.8	4%	2.6	29%*	3.4	8%*
Cerebrovascular diseases	2.1	– 7%*	0.3	3%	1.6	– 7%
including stroke	0.4	9%	0.2	34%	– 0.3	12%
Diseases of arteries and arterioles	2.2	0%	0.7	– 5%	1.7	– 2%
Venous and lymphatic diseases	7.6	6%*	4.1	– 6%*	6.5	3%*
All cardiovascular diseases	32.8	– 1%	11.5	4%*	26.3	– 1%*

Reading: 13.4 of every 100 general practitioner sessions in 1995-1996 were devoted to patients with hypertension. Since any given patient could have been suffering from several cardiovascular diseases, the entry for "all cardiovascular diseases" should not be interpreted as the percentage of sessions involving at least one cardiovascular disease. The variations marked with an asterisk(*) indicate a 95% significant difference in the raw data between 1992 and 1996.

Source: CREDES, EPPM-IMS France surveys 1991-1992/1995-1996.

Mental health

In France, mental health disorders affect millions of people to varying degrees, either personally or others with whom they come into contact; in the last few years, health professionals have made every effort to communicate more effectively with the general public, with the aim of informing, facilitating the recognition of mental health problems, and improving the image of mental illness. Depression, malaise among the young, and autism in children are all subjects which are gradually coming up for public discussion. Others, in spite of their gravity or frequency, such as schizophrenia or alcohol-related mental health problems, still too often go unrecognized.

In the domain of mental health, the 1994 HCSP report fixed two types of target, one related to chronic mental illness, and the other to depression and suicide.

Chronic psychiatric disorders

There is a lack of comparable surveys carried out on a regular basis, making it difficult to evaluate whether any targeted improvement in quality of life and social insertion of chronically ill patients has taken place. However, a certain number of changes have occurred.

Teams in the psychiatric sectors have changed their mode of intervention.

In 1995, almost 920,000 adults were managed by the psychiatric sectors – this corresponds to 22 patients followed-up per thousand inhabitants aged 20 years and over; between 1989 and 1995, there was a 30% increase in the number of patients being treated, primarily related to an appreciable rise in the number of those monitored as outpatients (+ 39%): almost 780,000 patients, *i.e.* 8 out of 10, were managed as outpatients in 1995.

The decline in full-time hospitalisation capacity is continuing: the number of beds per sector dropped from 94 in 1989 to 69 in 1995; however, the number of patients treated full-time rose by 10% from 1989 to 1995, with a reduction in the mean duration of the patient's stay. Nowadays, compulsory admissions account for only 11% of full-time hospitalisations. Between 1989 and 1995, the greatest increase (+ 73%) occurred in the number of patients treated on a part-time basis, but they occupy a modest place in the active stream of patients (11%).

It should be noted that while the active stream was continuously increasing, medical personnel remained stable between 1991 and 1995, with 6.4 full-time equivalents per sector, whereas non medical personnel tended to decline, dropping from 86.8 to 83.6 full-time equivalents per sector.

The patients' living conditions and bodily health have been described in a study of a cohort of 3,470 schizophrenic patients[16] (INSERM, Groupe français d'épidémiologie psychiatrique) which showed that most of them had social protection and access to physical treatment in 1995; they took considerable advantage of physical treatment, to a similar extent as that found among the general population. Moreover, *"the study confirmed, as others in France have done, that by providing treatment continuity, the policy of division into sectors produces relative protection from excessive exclusion"*[17].

To illustrate this opinion, it may be noted that a national survey in 1996, following on from the 1995 DGS report on "L'Évolution des soins en psychiatrie and la réinsertion des malades mentaux" (Changes in psychiatric treatment and reintegration of the mentally ill), identified 150 work initiatives in partnership leading to over 50 networks which contribute to the professional insertion of the mentally ill.

Nevertheless, the cohort of schizophrenic patients was monitored for two years and considerable excess mortality was found to have occurred:
– death due to natural causes among the patients was approximately twice as high as among the general population,
– the mortality rate due to suicide was excessively high – about twenty times higher among the schizophrenic patients than in the general population.

Thus, both users and professionals currently recognize that the target must be to improve the quality of life and social insertion of the chronically mentally ill; however, a review of the present situation shows that the measures so far adopted have not gone far enough.

While the principles of division into sectors are confirmed by these observations, there are differences in their implementation due, on the one hand, to psychiatric practices and the resources allocated and, on the other hand, to the diversity of the community's response to the social treatment of reinsertion. The present limits of management are clearly apparent in the excess mortality noted among patients, an indicator which will have to come under attentive scrutiny in the future.

---

16. Casadebaig F., et al., *"État somatique et accès aux soins de patients schizophrènes en secteur de psychiatrie générale"* (Physical condition and access to medical care of schizophrenic patients in general psychiatry), L'information psychiatrique, 1995, 3, 267-271.
17. Casadebaig F., Guilloud-Bataille J.M., Philippe A., *"Schizophrénie et exclusion sociale"* (Schizophrenia and social exclusion), Revue française de psychiatrie et psychologie médicale, 1997; 9: 25-28.

Part two Changes in health status

Mortality due to suicide Up until the middle of the 1980s, there was a continuous increase in the comparative suicide rate in France. It reached 23 per 100,000 in 1985, then declined up until 1991, remained stationary at above 20 per 100,000 and, with 11,300 deaths, stood at 19.5 per 100,000 in 1996. Thus, the general trend since 1985 has been a fall in the mortality rate due to suicide. However, a sharper decrease will be necessary to attain the target rate of 18 per 100,000 by the year 2000 (figure 24).

Figure 24 **Mortality due to suicide**
(comparative rates smoothed over 3-year periods)

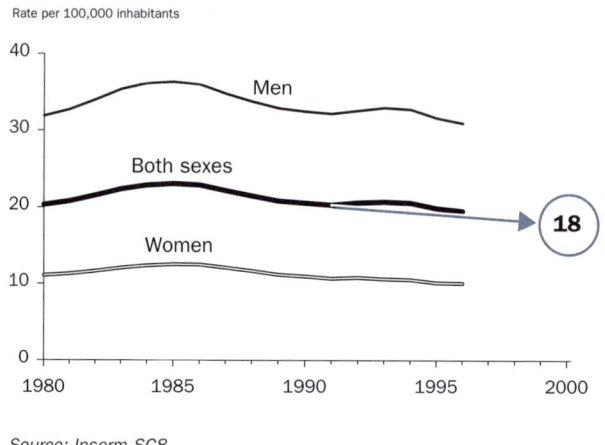

Source: Inserm SC8.

Suicide accounts for 2.2% of total deaths (3.1% and 1.3% of male and female deaths respectively), but is a substantial cause of premature mortality: within 25 years, the proportion of premature mortality attributable to suicide has doubled. An analysis of comparative mortality rates due to suicide by sex and by age groups shows that the highest rates were found among those 75 and over, and that the sharp increases in the suicide rate were particularly noted among men aged 25-44 between 1975 and 1996 (rising from 21.8 to 37.1). Among 15-24-year-olds during the same periods, the rate rose from 11.5 to 14.5 in men and dropped from 4.7 to 4.3 in women, making suicide the second cause of mortality after road accidents in this age group.

An inter-regional study covering the years 1992-1994 revealed notable differences: in Brittany, Lower Normandy, Picardy and Nord-Pas-de-Calais, the comparative mortality index revealed excess mortality rates of about 25% to almost 60% in these regions, similar to those noted in 1991-1993.

One study[18] carried out by five Regional Health Surveillance Centres (Aquitaine, Brittany, Midi-Pyrénées, Nord-Pas-de-Calais, Rhône-Alpes) estimated the annual number of attempted suicide patients admitted to hospital at 153,000. In 1993, an estimate by the "Service des statistiques, des études et des systèmes d'information" (SESI) (Statistics and Information Systems Department) put the number at 164,000. The report on suicide attempts and suicide-related deaths quoted a mean of 13, with variations from less than 9 in Brittany to almost 15 in the Nord-Pas-de-Calais and Rhône-Alpes regions. Moreover, a further survey reckoned that fewer than two in ten suicide attempts did not end in hospital admission. Several epidemiological studies have investigated the factors associated with the risk of suicide and repeated attempts, in addition to age, sex, socioprofessional category, marital status, and region of residence. The weight of individual psychopathological factors, the inadequacy of medical management following a failed first attempt, and the importance of family factors were all stressed.

Depression All of the above data underline the importance of the early detection of depressive disorders among the general population, as in those who attempt suicide.

Studies have recently been made of the prevalence of depressive states in the population: in the future, they should make it possible to discover any trends over time. Efforts have been made to standardise the methodology and this should facilitate comparison of the various countries which has so far not been possible.

The Depres *(Depression research in European society)* survey which has just been carried out in six European countries set itself the aim of determining the prevalence of depression over a 6-month period and the repercussions of depressive disorders on the general population; it involved more than 78,000 adults (including 15,000 in France) questioned using a standardised tool adapted to the screening of depression.

The 6-month results[19] indicate that the prevalence of depressive symptoms is 17%, including 6.9% major depression, each individual country showing differences, with France and the United Kingdom in first place (9.1%). Major depression occurs predominantly in women (*sex ratio* 2:1 in France), though the rates for minor depression are equivalent in the two sexes. The study estimated that one third of subjects with major depression failed to seek help for their disorders; on the other hand, they frequently con-

---

18. ORS (Regional Health Surveillance Centres) Aquitaine, Bretagne, Midi-Pyrénées, Nord-Pas-de-Calais, Rhône-Alpes, *"Prévention des suicides et tentatives de suicide: État des lieux"* (Prevention of suicide and attempted suicide: status report), Paris, Association Premutam, 1998, 317 p.
19. Lépine J.P., Gatspar M., Mendlewicz J., Tylee A. *Depression in the community: the first pan European study Depres.* Int Clin Psychopharmacol, 1997; 12: 19-29.

Part two Changes in health status

sulted a doctor – but for other reasons: the mean number of consultations over the 6-month period was 3 times higher for those presenting with major depression compared with subjects who were not depressed.

This last observation confirms the estimates made by CREDES showing that, for depressed subjects, medical care consumption over three months was three times higher than that of unaffected subjects (over 3,600 F *versus* 1,200 F), whereas the cost of treatment for depressive illness over the same period was put at 790 F (CREDES 1996).

All these indications point to the fact that the diagnosis of depression must be improved and its treatment not merely restricted to the administration of a drug, but rather conceived in terms of overall management involving both GPs and specialists.

The perinatal period and first year of life

Changes in infantile mortality

During the 1990s, the infantile mortality rate showed a spectacular drop in France: from 7.3‰ in 1990 to 4.9‰ in 1995 and 4.8‰ in 1996; the rate for 1997 climbed slightly back over the mark of five per thousand (5.1‰) but remained well below the 1994 level (5.9‰). While there is a general downward trend in developed countries, it was particularly accentuated during this period in France where the situation is markedly improving relative to other countries – France now comes just after the Nordic countries (Finland, Norway: 4‰; Sweden: 4.1‰) and Japan (4.3‰), and ahead of Germany, the Netherlands and Canada – all countries which had a lower infantile mortality rate in 1990 (figure 25).

The general target set in the 1994 HCSP report of reducing mortality by 20% by the year 2000 has been greatly exceeded where infantile mortality is concerned.

Almost half the drop has occurred thanks to the decrease in mortality due to sudden infant death syndrome. The latter was the cause of 1,369 deaths in 1990 and only 538 in 1995, the figures for total deaths being 5,599 and 3,545 respectively.

Because of this, the decade of the 1990s is marking a break with earlier decades in terms of the structure of infantile mortality which, during the 1970s and 1980s, saw a drop that was actually due to a reduction in the number of early deaths (neonatal mortality[20])

---

20. Neonatal mortality rate: the number of infants who die between birth and 27 days post partum per thousand live births.
It is divided into: early neonatal mortality (0-7 days) and late neonatal mortality (8-27 days).

Figure 25 **Variation in infantile mortality rate**

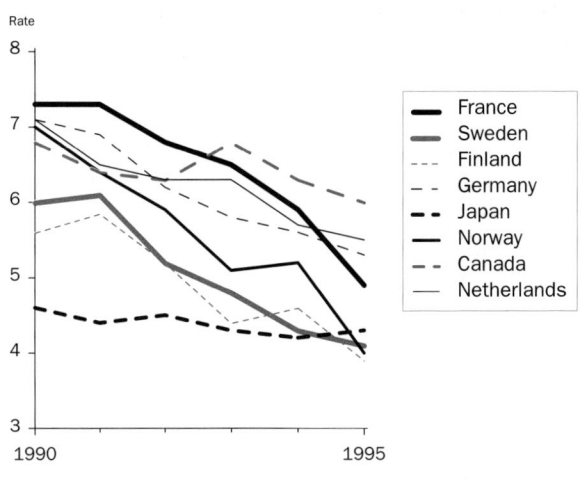

Source: OECD.

whereas post-neonatal mortality[21] (the period during which sudden death syndrome occurs) remained unchanged (table 32). Conversely, it was the drop in post-neonatal mortality which accounted for two thirds of the total reduction during the period 1990-1996.

In addition to sudden death syndrome, the principal causes of death before one year are a group of conditions arising in the perinatal period (one third) and congenital abnormalities (one quarter). Of the first group, respiratory distress syndrome and other respiratory disorders have decreased by 35%, while deaths due to congenital abnormalities have fallen by 25%.

Inter-regional differences in infantile mortality remained high during recent periods, with rates ranging from 7 to 7.6‰ in northern France to 5.4 to 5.7‰ in the south-east and west. There has been very little change in the respective order of the infantile mortality rate in the regions.

In the course of the last two decades, the infantile mortality rate fell considerably in French overseas territories (except in Guyana) to the point where it approached levels in France. However, stabilisation and even slight regression has been noted in this indicator during the 1990s, except in the case of Martinique which achieved rates below those of fifteen or so French departments.

---

21. Postneonatal mortality rate: the number of infants who die between 28 and 365 days post partum per thousand live births.

Changes in perinatal mortality

Perinatal mortality – which encompasses not only infant deaths recorded within 7 days of birth but also stillborn infants – decreased from 8.3‰ in 1990 to 7.4‰ in 1996, thanks to an appreciable retreat between 1991 and 1992; the rate has been constant since 1994 (table 32).

Table 32 **Variation in the different components of infantile mortality between 1970 and 1997 in France**

	Infantile mortality rate	Infantile mortality components Mortality			Perinatal mortality rate
		Early neonatal	Neonatal	Post-neonatal	
1970	18.2	10.2	12.6	5.5	23.3
1975	13.8	7.3	9.2	4.7	18.1
1980	10.0	4.4	5.8	4.3	12.9
1985	8.3	3.4	4.6	3.7	10.7
1990	7.3	2.5	3.6	3.8	8.3
1991	7.3	2.5	3.5	3.8	8.2
1992	6.8	2.3	3.3	3.5	7.7
1993	6.5	2.2	3.1	3.3	7.5
1994	5.9	2.3	3.2	2.7	7.4
1995	4.9	2.2	2.9	2.0	7.4
1996	4.8[a]	2.2[a]	3.0[a]	1.8[a]	7.4[a]
1997	5.1[a]				

a. Provisional data.

The target of 6.5‰ by the year 2000 given in the 1994 HCSP report and the governmental perinatal plan devised in the same year is attainable as long as there is a very rapid resumption of the decline (figure 26).

France's position relative to countries with a similar level of development is less favourable in terms of perinatal than infantile mortality, since the stillbirth rate is higher by one to two per thousand (France is in about tenth position). Between 1990 and 1995, the perinatal mortality rate dropped in many countries to the same extent that it had fallen in France: hence, France's position remained stable over this period.

Western regions have the lowest rates (between 5.9 and 6.4‰), the mean for France as a whole being 7.5. The regions with the highest rates are more scattered (Corsica, Languedoc-Roussillon, Picardy, Franche-Comté, Limousin, Champagne-Ardenne). The situation is getting worse in Burgundy, Poitou-Charentes and Lorraine, while it is improving in the Auvergne and Nord-Pas-de-Calais.

Overseas territories with the best results (Martinique and Réunion) have rates consistently more than 50% higher than the French mean, making their level equivalent to that in France at the start

Indicators of health status

of the 1980s. The rate in Guadeloupe is twice that recorded in France, placing it at the same level as France twenty years ago. The situation in Guyana is particularly serious: the perinatal mortality rate is close to 30‰ and, above all, has shown no improvement in the last ten years or so.

Figure 26 **Perinatal mortality**
(rates smoothed per 1,000 live births)

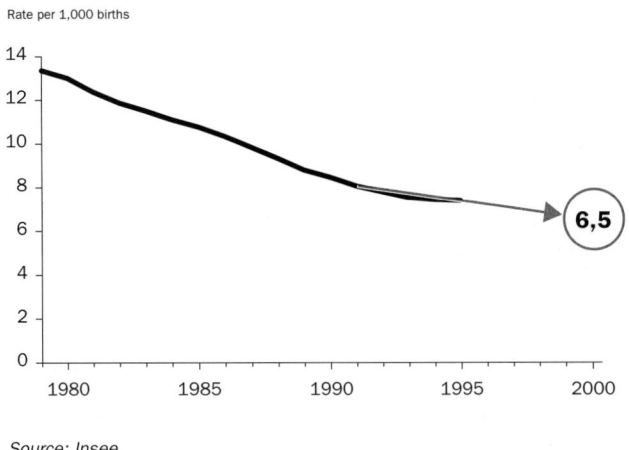

Source: Insee.

Changes in maternal mortality

Cases of maternal death have become rare in developed countries (about ten or so cases per 100,000 births). The level of maternal mortality is regarded as a highly significant factor in the health of a community.

Over the last two decades, a regular decline was noted up until 1989, followed by an increase up until 1992, and then fluctuations around the level that had been achieved (figure 27). These unfavourable changes since 1990 probably result from the better quality of information collected. The alternative hypothesis – that the rates reflect poorer quality in medical care – cannot be entirely excluded, but would contradict changes that have taken place amongst the other indicators of the perinatal period.

It is difficult to make international comparisons because of problems involved in notification. However, a comparison with countries known to have reliable systems for pinpointing maternal deaths (Scandinavian countries, United Kingdom) clearly shows that the number of maternal deaths is high in France and that a large number of such deaths could be avoided.

Regardless of the difficulties in interpretation related to problems of death certification, it would seem that the current trend will fall

Part two   Changes in health status

short of the targeted 30% reduction in maternal mortality set out in the 1994 governmental perinatal plan and also in the 1994 HCSP report.

Figure 27 **Maternal mortality**
(number of deaths not smoothed)

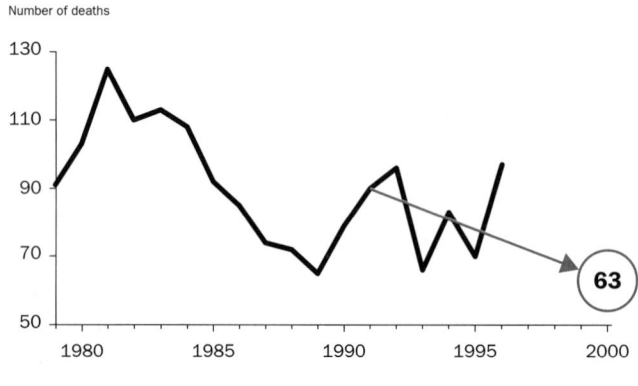

Source: Inserm SC8.

Changes in the frequency of prematurity and low birth weight

Given that considerable progress has been made in terms of mortality, it is becoming increasingly important to appreciate the quality of life of the survivors. From this point of view, two problems dominate perinatal morbidity, *i.e.* prematurity and low birth weight (dysmaturity). Both are not only essential risk factors in mortality, but also give rise to handicaps and death at a later age.

The most recent general data derive from the January 1995 national perinatal survey which indicated that there had been no reduction in these indicators. Over a 15-year period, the prematurity rate (birth before 37 weeks' gestation) remained stable for all births: 6.0% in 1981, when the previous general survey was carried out, and 5.9% in 1995. The proportion of very premature infants (born before 34 weeks) rose from 1.1% to 1.6%, while that of infants with low birth weight (less than 2500 g) increased from 5.2% to 6.2% – the rise among infants with very low birth weight (less than 1,500 g) was particularly pronounced (from 0.4% to 1.1%).

Considering live births only, the rates for prematurity and marked prematurity were respectively 5.4% and 1.2% in 1995; the proportion of infants born live weighing less than 2,500 g was 5.7% and that of infants born live weighing less than 1,500 g was 0.7%.

High Committee on Public Health

Taking 730,000 as the annual number of births, these rates represent about 43,000 premature births every year, including 12,000 very premature births and, among live births, between 39,000 and 40,000 premature infants including 9,000 very premature infants.

According to the Apgar score[22], the health status of infants at birth remained stable from 1981 to 1995. 2.2% of live infants had a score of less than five at one minute (1.8% in 1981) and 1.5% had a score of less than eight at five minutes, which may be regarded as a criterion of neonatal distress (1.6% in 1981).

One survey carried out in 1988-1989 in certain regions of France showed that although the prematurity rate started to fall during the 1980s from 6.5 to 4.8% and then rose again to 5.6% in 1995, births of infants weighing less than 2,500 g increased from 5.3% in 1981 to 5.7% in 1988-1989 and stayed at this level in 1995. Births of very low birth weight infants (less than 1,500 g) increased steadily throughout the period (from 0.2 to 0.5, then 0.7%). These results confirmed earlier studies which had shown that the perinatal policy adopted since the beginning of the 1970s had brought about progress in terms of prematurity but had only had a relative effect in improving the birth weight.

Multiple pregnancies made a large contribution to premature births. The prematurity rate was eight times higher for twins than for singleton births; in fact, 41% of twins were born prematurely. Multiple births accounted for 2.7% of all births, but 17% of premature births and 20% of births where the infant weighed less than 2,500 g. Thus, the prematurity rate dropped from 5.4% for all live births to 4.5% among live singleton births.

Because of modifications in obstetric practice, infants who are threatened *in utero* tend to be delivered earlier and earlier, thereby contributing to an increase in the rate of premature and underweight infants. Thus, 42% of infants under 35 weeks and 50% of infants weighing less than 2,000 g were born after a medical decision has been taken to interrupt the pregnancy by caesarean section or induction of labour. Consequently, an increase in very premature or underweight infants does not necessarily indicate that the long-term prognosis for such infants is worse. The results from ongoing studies on the fate of very premature infants must be awaited before the long-term consequences of these decisions are known.

Recent changes in the social situation of women in France might produce different outcomes. On the one hand, better prevention

---

22. Every neonate undergoes a complete examination at the time of birth.
    The Apgar score is determined by assessing the following five components assigned 1 or 2 points each: heart rate, respiratory effort, muscle tone, reflex irritability, and skin colour.
    The Apgar score assessed at five minutes after birth provides information as to the infant's adaptation to extra-uterine life.

may result from the higher average level of training and in the percentage of women who are employed. At the same time, prenatal monitoring has been increased so that in 1995, 17.2% of women had 7 prenatal visits, *i.e.* the mandatory number if delivery occurs at term, and 73.3% more than 7 visits – the corresponding figure in 1981 was 42.5%. Women are more frequently prepared for delivery, especially if it is their first child (64.5% in 1995 *versus* 50.6% in 1981).

On the other hand, increasing vulnerability and isolation tend to produce less prenatal monitoring and an increase in risk factors. Thus, 32% of women without any stated resources had fewer than 7 prenatal visits compared with 19.5% of women who had various financial aids (subsidy, allowance, minimum welfare benefits), and only 7.5% of those who earned their living. In terms of the outcome of pregnancy, 13.5% of women with no stated means had a premature infant compared with 7.5% of those with various financial aids and 5.5% of those with an income from working.

Handicaps and dependency

Many epidemiological and statistical data concerning handicaps and dependency are available but they are disparate and have large gaps, making it particularly difficult to identify changes in relevant indicators over time in this field.

The survey on handicaps, disability and dependency (HDD) presented below will be an important step in making the information system uniform in this domain and suitable as a point of reference for later trends.

Changes in the employment rate among handicapped people and work in a sheltered environment

The target set by the 1994 HCSP report was to improve the quality of life and social integration of people needing help with the activities of daily life. No assessment can be made of changes in the quality of life due to a lack of suitable indicators; at the most, it can be noted that progress is still being made far too slowly in terms of important factors such as accessible transportation and the spread of temporary replacement services for help in day-to-day living.

On the other hand, it is possible to monitor changes in the employment of handicapped people. The employment of handicapped individuals in an ordinary environment is growing but the legal requirement of 6% handicapped employees has never been attained (table 33): it is currently slightly over 4%. It should be noted that about 20% of companies, frequently of a considerable size, satisfy their legal obligations by signing subcontracting agreements with companies that provide a sheltered working environment.

Table 33 **Number of handicapped persons employed by firms with at least 20 employees**
(private sector establishments with 20 employees or more, as a percentage)

	Number of handicapped persons employed	Employment rate
1989	235,000	3.58
1990	236,000	3.72
1991	258,000	3.76
1992	254,700	4.00
1993	254,500	4.06
1994	247,900	4.11
1995[a]	266,000	4.12

a. In 1995, the file of establishments used as the base in the survey was modified. Hence, the number of handicapped workers employed cannot be compared directly with the number in previous years. However, the 4.12% employment rate was calculated relative to a constant base of establishments.
Source: DARES, Survey of the obligation to employ handicapped workers, 1995.

In companies with fewer than twenty employees, the rate of employment of handicapped workers was estimated to be 1.1% of the work force, *i.e.* 50,000.

In the civil service in 1994, the number of those taking advantage of obligatory employment was 72,370 out of a total of 2,296,500 state employees, *i.e.* the handicapped employment rate was 3.15% on 31 December 1994, having slightly progressed with respect to previous results (2.9% in 1993 and 3% in 1992)[23].

It is impossible to integrate some of the handicapped directly and immediately into an ordinary company and they must then be oriented towards special organisations: CATs ("centres d'aide par le travail" or Disabled Persons Workshops) and sheltered workshops.

In 1995, 1,284 CATs had about 83,700 places available and 382 sheltered workshops had 13,400 places, with an occupation rate of almost 100%. Since 1983, the mean annual increase in the number of handicapped persons working in CATs has been 3.8%, and that in sheltered workshops has been 11% over the same period (although, it must be said, the initial work force was much smaller in the latter) (table 34).

---

23. These data concerning the employment of handicapped persons only include those employed within the framework of the law of 1987. It is likely that other individuals who might be classifiable as handicapped are not counted, either because they have not approached a COTOREP, or because they did not wish to draw attention to their situation.

Part two — Changes in health status

Table 34 **Variation in capacity of disabled persons workshops and sheltered workshops during the period 1983-1995**

	Disabled persons workshops		Sheltered workshops	
	N. of establishments	N. of places	N. of establishments	N. of places
1983	809	53,430	62	3,856
1985	911	58,297	106	5,369
1987	999	64,751	137	6,532
1989	1,065	68,513	180	7,906
1991	1,123	73,576	268	9,813
1993	1,216	78,849	306	11,433
1995	1,284	83,666	382	13,446

Source: SESI ES surveys.

It should be noted that work in a sheltered environment was originally designed to provide a temporary transition period prior to integration in an ordinary environment; in actual practice, these structures have become specific work places. In fact, in 1994, fewer than 1% of workers left their CAT for an ordinary environment or sheltered workshop; and it has been estimated that, in 1990, 3% of handicapped employees left sheltered workshops for an ordinary environment.

Degrees of handicap and dependency

Using as a basis various sources dating from 1991 (decennial health survey) to 1997 (recipients of allocations), a few figures can be quoted that give an idea of the size of the health problem.

In 1991, 5,480,000 person living at home declared a handicap or needed help in daily life, and 940,000 received specific cash benefits. 430,000 persons over the age of 65 were bedridden or confined to an armchair or needed assistance in washing and dressing.

In medical and welfare establishments in 1996, 278,000 persons were living in an institution or were being cared for by a specialised home care service, including 79,000 adults in lodgings and 125,000 children.

376,800 dependent persons were living in retirement homes and long-stay facilities in 1994, including 360,000 aged 65 and over.

The most recent description of the distribution of deficits among the handicapped population living at home comes from the 1991 decennial health survey whose results were already quoted in the 1994 HCSP report. In this, the mean number of deficits declared per 100 persons was 10, ranging from 2.6 in those under 20, to 6.8 between 20 and 60 years, and to 27.4 in persons over 60. Motor deficits were the most common deficit among the elderly, whereas failing eyesight which could not be effectively compensated was most frequent among those under 60. Failings in mental and intellectual capacities were less common (respectively 0.6

and 0.5% among the entire population). However, those subjects who presented such failings received financial assistance more often than the others. Similarly, many more of them received regular help in their daily lives, and half of them were officially recognized as handicapped by aid organisations.

Those with motor deficits most often sought help in moving around but less financial assistance than those with psychiatric or intellectual disorders.

Those with failing eyesight and, to a lesser extent, hearing loss, stand out sharply from others with a declared handicap or disability in daily life. Those with poor eyesight are more autonomous and benefit less than other handicapped individuals from available daily living assistance. They also receive less failing-related financial aid, and rarely require regular assistance or help in getting about. Failing eyesight is, according to the vast majority of replies given in the survey, a handicap which allows a relatively normal life, even though it does create some difficulties.

THE HID (HANDICAPS, INCAPACITÉS, DÉPENDANCE) SURVEY

The HID (handicaps, disability and dependency) survey is being conducted by the "Institut national de la statistique et des études économiques" (INSEE) (National Institute for Economic Studies and Statistics) in co-operation with the "Service des statistiques et des systèmes d'information" (SESI) (Statistics and Information Systems Department), the "Mission recherche expérimentation" (MIRE) (Task Force on Research and Experimentation) of the Ministry of Employment and Solidarity, and the "Centre de recherche et d'études en économie de la santé" (CREDES) (Centre for Research and Documentation on Health Economics).

It has three objectives: to determine the number of dependent persons; to evaluate the fluctuation in disablement (onset and termination of disability); and to note the nature, quantity and existing providers of assistance, as well as unsatisfied needs. The survey has to cover all types of situation, *i.e.* persons who live at home, in an institution and, if possible, those without a home.

As far as people living at home are concerned, it became apparent that 20,000 persons would need to be questioned for the sample and this extensive operation will be inserted into the next general census of the population in March 1999.

Data concerning fluctuations among the disabled are required for the setting up of studies designed to predict variations in the number of individuals having handicaps with differing degrees of severity: they will be obtained by re-questioning the subjects after a two year interval.

The survey among persons living in an institution will take place in October 1998, with a sample size of 15,000, and the first results should be available at the end of 1999. The questioning will be repeated in the year 2000 for these persons.

The regions or departments will be given the possibility of extending this national operation.

Part two Changes in health status

Back pain

The target set by the 1994 general report, *Health in France*, was to *"reduce the frequency and gravity of back pain, especially severe lower back pain, which is incapacitating and can cause social alienation"*.

Two types of indicator have been adopted in monitoring changes in this disorder, *i.e.* spinal problems declared during surveys of households, and the frequency of sessions with a doctor because of such problems.

The latest health and social protection surveys for the periods 1988-1991 and 1992-1995 revealed that most spinal problems were relatively stable, apart from the rate of declaration of arthritis and inflammatory conditions which rose from 3.7 to 5.9% (table 35).

Within four years, from 1991-1992 to 1995-1996, the number of sessions for spinal problems rose from 43 to 48 per thousand sessions for all doctors combined, and from 52 to 58 per thousand sessions among GPs. The increased incidence of spinal problems primarily concerned the "cervical vertebrae" group (+ 26%) and the "slipped disk, low back pain, sciatica" group (+ 14%). Extrapolated over the whole year, this meant that the total number of doctor sessions for this disorder increased from 12.8 to 16.2 million, *i.e.* an augmentation of 27%, twice as high as the increase in the total number of sessions between the two periods (+ 13%).

Table 35 **Prevalence of spinal conditions**
(as a percentage)

	1988-1991	1992-1995
Spinal conditions	12.3	14.6
Including		
Slipped disk, low back pain, sciatica	7.7	8.0
Arthritis and inflammatory conditions	3.7	5.9
Kyphoscoliosis	0.6	0.5
Cervical involvement (other than arthritis)	0.3	0.3

Reading: 8.0% of individuals suffered from a slipped disk, low back pain or sciatica in 1992-1995, while the corresponding figure in 1988-1991 was 7.7%.
Source: ESPS surveys 1988-1991 and 1992-1995.

Thus, declarations of spinal problems are relatively stable, but those affected seek help from their doctors far more frequently (table 36).

Table 36 **Consultation of a doctor in private practice for a spinal condition**
(rate per 100 sessions)

	All doctors in private practice		General practitioners	
	1996	Variation 1992-1996	1996	Variation 1992-1996
Spinal conditions	48.0	12%	57.9	11%
Including				
Slipped disk, low back pain, sciatica	32.5	14%	40.4	12%
Arthritis and inflammatory conditions	6.0	– 7%	6.4	– 9%
Kyphoscoliosis	1.1	– 4%	1.3	– 1%
Cervical involvement (other than arthritis)	8.4	26%	9.8	25%
Number of sessions per year (in millions)	16.2	13.6		
Variation 1992-1996	27%	24%		

Source: CREDES, EPPM-IMS France survey 1991-1992 and 1995-1996.

Sexually transmitted diseases

HIV infection and AIDS

Since the start of the AIDS epidemic and as of 31 December 1997, 48,396 cases of AIDS had been notified in France; of these, 29,737 (61%) have died (data corrected for lag time to notification). Taking into account deaths which have not been notified, the total number of deaths due to AIDS in France since the beginning of the epidemic is probably more in the region of 35,000 to 37,000. The number of living people infected with AIDS was estimated at between 19,000 and 21,000 as of 31 December 1997.

Sharp drop in the incidence of AIDS since 1996

Both the introduction of powerful new therapeutic antiviral combinations (triple therapies) in 1995 and their subsequent widespread use in 1996 led to a sudden decrease in the incidence of AIDS in France in 1996 (figure 28).

This drop – unprecedented in the history of the AIDS epidemic – continued in 1997. In 1995, 5,208 new cases of AIDS and 3,876 AIDS-related deaths were recorded, compared with 2,289 cases and 1,311 deaths in 1997 (numbers corrected for 1997 lag time to notification). An analysis of the causes which might explain this sudden drop ruled out any bias linked to a delay in notification, or a revised definition of AIDS in 1993, or a decrease in the incidence of infection in previous years, making it reasonable to attribute the 56% reduction in incidence and 66% reduction in the mortality rate over 2 years to the utilisation of novel treatments. In the 3 main transmission groups, the number of new AIDS cases has fallen, though the general trend is different for each group.

Part two Changes in health status

Figure 28 **Number of cases of AIDS per 6-month diagnosis period**
(data corrected for lag time to notification, 31 December 1997)

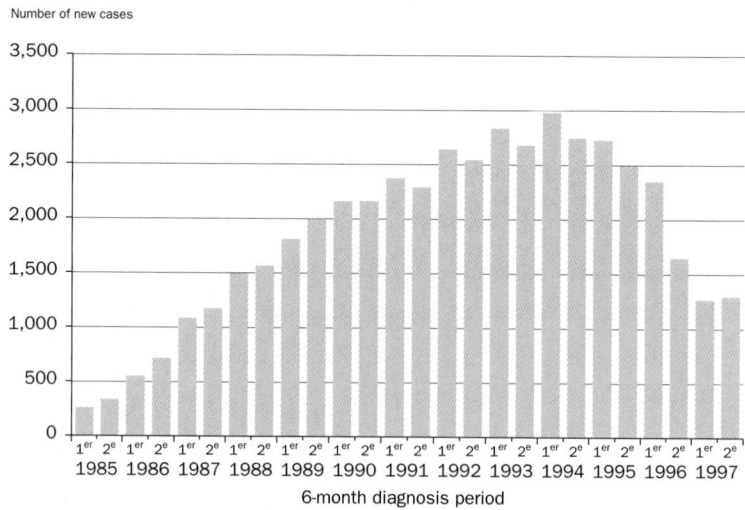

Source: RNSP.

Among homosexuals, the decrease noted in 1996 was actually an accentuation of the decline which had started in mid-1994; among intravenous drug users, the sudden drop in the 2nd quarter of 1996 followed a period of stabilisation between 1992 and 1995; among heterosexuals, the number of cases of AIDS increased up until 1995 and then fell in 1996. The tendency to decline persisted in 1997, without becoming more pronounced (– 15% between the two half-year periods). In all, a decrease of over 40% occurred in the number of cases between 1996 and 1997 (55% among drug addicts, 46% among homosexuals and bisexuals, and 30% among the heterosexuals).

The patient population which develops full-blown AIDS consists of 3 subpopulations: subjects who were unaware that they were seropositive before AIDS became apparent (and who have therefore not benefited from pre-AIDS antiretroviral therapy), subjects who knew that they were seropositive before developing AIDS but were untreated, and subjects who knew beforehand that they were seropositive and had been treated (figure 29).

The distribution of the 3 groups over the period 1994 to mid-1996 shows that it remained stable over time (22% did not know their serologic status, 23% knew they were seropositive but remained untreated, and 55% had received antiretroviral therapy prior to developing AIDS). This breakdown of the AIDS population under-

Figure 29 **New cases of AIDS per 6-month diagnosis period as a function of whether patients knew they were seropositive and whether antiretroviral therapy had been prescribed before they developed AIDS**
(corrected data, 31 December 1997)

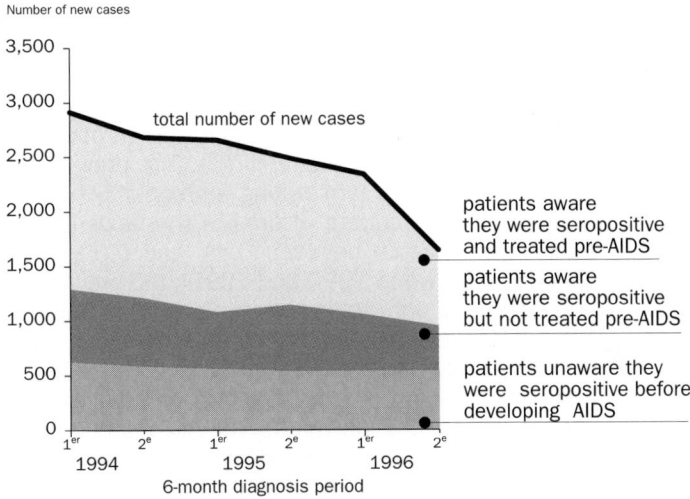

Source: RNSP.

went a change when new antiretroviral combinations were introduced in 1996: in the last quarter of 1997, 46% of AIDS cases were unaware of their serologic status, 28% knew they were seropositive but had not taken antiretroviral agents before developing AIDS, and 24% knew and had taken antiretroviral agents pre-AIDS. This change indicates that the highly positive impact of new therapies is limited by inadequate early screening for HIV infection and also by inadequate or delayed management of patients who know that they are seropositive. In addition, it should be stressed that at the stage of full-blown AID, the subjects' non-awareness of their HIV seropositivity – and hence the impact of novel therapies – depends on the at-risk group to which they belong: in the 2nd quarter of 1997, 56% of heterosexuals, 45% of homosexuals and bisexuals, and 20% of intravenous drug users did not know they were HIV positive. Among heterosexuals and intravenous drug users, fewer men than women knew they were seropositive at the time of AIDS diagnosis (64% of heterosexual men *versus* 46% of heterosexual women, and 22% of male drug addicts *versus* 10% of female drug addicts).

Part two Changes in health status

The detection of subjects infected by HIV and early management are essential in the fight against AIDS

The prevalence of HIV infection in France has been estimated by various methods, *i.e.* modelling using retroactive calculations or simulations, and methods related to meta-analysis combining all the available data concerning HIV infection in France. In 1994, its prevalence was estimated at approximately 110,000 cases. Anonymous surveys which eliminate any participation bias linked to knowledge of seropositivity status have also been carried out every two years in two French regions (Île-de-France and Provence-Alpes-Côte-d'Azur) among pregnant women and among a national sample of venereal disease clinics. The prevalence of HIV infection among women terminating a pregnancy had not appreciably altered over the course of time in the Île-de-France region (variation in prevalence between 0.4% and 0.5% for the 4 surveys conducted between 1990 and 1996); the prevalence of HIV infection increased only among women over 35 – this result is consistent with the ageing noted among seropositive patients detected in other studies. In the PACA region, HIV prevalence among pregnant women showed no change over time. Among patients attending VD clinics, the prevalence of HIV infection was also stable between 1991 and 1995. However, an analysis by age group showed that HIV infection had become less prevalent among consulting patients under 25 years of age and more prevalent among homosexuals aged 35 and over.

Based on a comparison of prevalence data and data from a survey on "problems and services required by persons infected by HIV", the population affected by HIV in France can be broken down as follows: 80,000 seropositive persons under management, and 30,000 persons undetected or detected but not under management.

No accurate information is available concerning the incidence of HIV infection. However, indirect estimates have been obtained by using data derived from repeated surveys of prevalence among pregnant women in the Île-de-France region and by taking mortality and fertility into account. The annual incidence among women of child-bearing age in the Île-de-France region has been estimated at 1.3‰ (95%-confidence interval: 0.51-2.05) over the period 1992-1993 and at 0.75‰ (confidence interval: 0.37-1.12) over the period 1990-1991.

There has been a regular decrease in the estimated annual number of subjects infected by HIV who discover that they are seropositive (from 24,423 in 1989 to 12,222 in 1996) with a parallel decrease in the rate of positive test results (0.97% in 1989 and 0.28% in 1996) (table 37).

Indicators of health status

In the Aquitaine region, data available for the various at-risk groups suggest that an increase occurred in the number of homosexuals/bisexuals and heterosexuals who discovered that they were seropositive in 1996 (figure 30). Moreover, an analysis of new HIV infections documented in various French information systems between 1991 and 1995 indicates that homosexuals and bisexuals are still the most affected group (representing 41% to 57% of the total), followed by heterosexuals (23% to 37%) and drug addicts (8% to 15%).

Table 37 **Variation in the estimated number of HIV seropositive individuals, in screening tests and in the seropositivity rate in Metropolitan France, Renavi, 1989-1996**

	N. of WB +	N. of serologic tests	Positivity rate (%)[a]
1989	24,423	2,507,248	0.97
1990	21,264	2,986,825	0.71
1991	19,540	3,474,234	0.56
1992	19,042	4,044,263	0.47
1993	16,449	4,704,020	0.35
1994	15,135	4,950,123	0.30
1995	13,766	4,832,855	0.28
1996	12,222	4,440,945	0.28

a. Positivity rate = Number of WB+/Number of serologic tests.
Source: RNSP.

Figure 30 **Annual number of patients in the Aquitaine region who discovered they were seropositive as a function of their transmission group from 1989 to 1997**

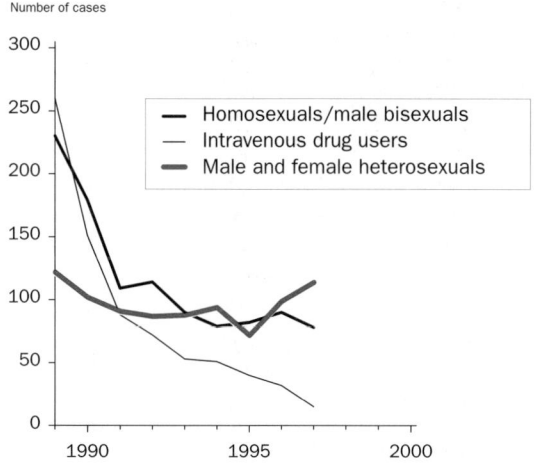

Source: ORS Aquitaine, 1997: provisional data.

Since the mid-1990s, attempts have been made to more clearly identify the HIV seropositive population in France, the characteristics of infected individuals, and screening and management modalities so that primary and secondary prevention programmes can be more effectively targeted. More recently, new treatment strategies have completely changed the natural history of the disease: this has been clearly shown by AIDS surveillance, and the modalities of AIDS management, even though the experience acquired so far has been limited. These favourable developments based on new therapies can only be extended if the subjects most exposed to risk are given easier access to HIV screening and early management. In fact, by the last quarter of 1997, there were still about 45% of AIDS cases which could not be avoided by early management (patients not known to be seropositive at the time of AIDS diagnosis), and about 28% of patients knew they were seropositive but were not taking pre-AIDS antiviral therapy. Unless there is a substantial decrease in these two high percentages in coming years, the reduction in the number of AIDS cases will not continue. In addition, surveillance must now be directed towards newly discovered HIV seropositive patients and their characteristics so as to tailor screening, management and prevention policy for maximum efficiency.

The incidence of the main sexually transmitted diseases in constant decline since 1986

Only gonococcal infections and genital chlamydial infections will be dealt with in this section. Infection by hepatitis B is sexually transmitted and will be treated in the following section. Other sexually transmitted diseases, especially syphilis, have become rare in France; however, a recrudescence of syphilis has recently been reported in eastern European countries and therefore deserves particular attention.

A network of laboratories (Renago) distributed throughout France is responsible for the surveillance of genital infections due to gonococci. Since 1986, the incidence of gonococcal infections has been decreasing (figure 31).

However, the reduction has slowed down for the past few years, especially among men. In 1996, 169 gonococcal infections were identified by Renago, men between 20 and 40 years of age being the most commonly affected (75%). Anorectal gonococcal infections increased among men between 1994 and 1995 and have since stabilised. The anorectal forms have been reported solely in the Île-de-France region and indicate that sexual practices involving a risk of HIV transmission still persist. Approximately 15% of gonococcal genital infections are acquired abroad (half in Africa and Asia). It should also be pointed out that gonococcal strains have developed chromosomally-determined resistance to penicillin and tetracycline since 1992.

Figure 31 **Variation in the mean number of strains of *N. gonorrhoeae* identified per year per laboratory, Renago from 1986 to 1996**

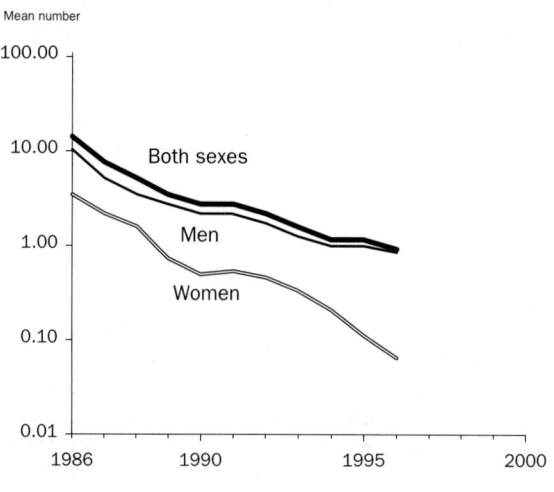

Source: RNSP.

Genital infections due to chlamydia are far more common than gonococcal infections, especially in women; they are monitored by a network of laboratories (Renachla) extending throughout France. In 1996, 1,494 chlamydial infections were identified by Renachla, including 1,061 in women. Renachla also indicated that the incidence of chlamydial infections has shown a regular decline since 1990 in men and women (56% decrease between 1990 and 1996 among men and 51% among women). Most patients are in the 20 to 34 age group (64%). The greater number of diagnoses in women does not automatically indicate an increased incidence – not only is the infection symptomatic in women far more often than in men, but there are far more frequent opportunities for detection among women. The clinical forms may have serious or even grave consequences for women, particularly salpingitis which is often responsible for secondary sterility. Given the repercussions of chlamydial infections on fertility, and the fact that ever more efficient diagnostic tests and effective treatments which avoid complications if used early enough are available, young women should be screened for chlamydial infections, particularly during regular gynaecological checkups (or if the woman's partner tests positive for *Chlamydia*).

The lower incidence of these 2 sexually transmitted diseases and present rarity of primary and secondary syphilis are indirect indicators that prevention programmes aimed at HIV infection have had an impact. Obviously, vigilance must be maintained, even though the incidence of these two diseases is at its lowest level ever.

Viral hepatitis Recent advances in our understanding of the epidemiology of the 3 main types of hepatitis (A, B and C) are analysed below. Hepatitis B and hepatitis C are primarily transmitted via blood: they both give rise to chronic liver disease and accordingly have a delayed adverse effect on morbidity, mortality and the medical care system. In addition, the interaction of these 2 chronic infections with excessive alcohol consumption is a major determinant in the incidence of cirrhosis of the liver and hence appreciable associated mortality (approximately 10,000 deaths due to cirrhosis every year in France).

Hepatitis A

Hepatitis A virus (HAV) is spread by the faecal-oral route, either from person to person or via contaminated food. Hepatitis A is an acute infection whose severity increases with age and which does not progress to a more chronic form. With the advances made in hygiene, the incidence of this infection has considerably decreased in France, especially among children and adolescents. This is illustrated by changes in the prevalence of anti-HAV antibodies (whose presence indicates previous infection) among national service conscripts: it dropped from 50% in 1978 to 10% in 1995. Given that immunity to the natural infection is life-long, adults are, and will be in the future, less and less protected by natural infection (frequently asymptomatic or not very severe in children and adolescents). The incidence of severe, especially fulminant, forms increases with age and, paradoxically, the serious morbidity related to this virus might increase. HAV infection among adults suffering from chronic liver disease (chronic hepatitis C in particular) is responsible for a far greater proportion of cases of fulminant hepatitis than among adults with a healthy liver.

The estimated incidence of acute hepatitis in France was 16 per 100,000 habitants in 1996 (*i.e.* about 9,000 new cases); in 1991, it was estimated at 27 per 100,000 (figure 32).

Its incidence according to age is bimodal, with a peak in children aged 5 to 14 years and another peak in young adults (20 to 40 years). The monthly distribution of new cases points to a recrudescence at the end of summer (September and October). The risk factors most commonly identified are travelling in southern countries, contact with a case of hepatitis A and, more rarely, possibly contaminated food.

A highly effective inactivated vaccine is now available and vaccine-induced immunity is probably very long-lasting. It is recommended for at-risk groups, especially for people travelling to countries where the disease is endemic. However, its present cost acts as a considerable deterrent to wider use.

Figure 32 **Incidence of symptomatic acute hepatitis A and B in France, 1991-1996**
(rate per 100,000)

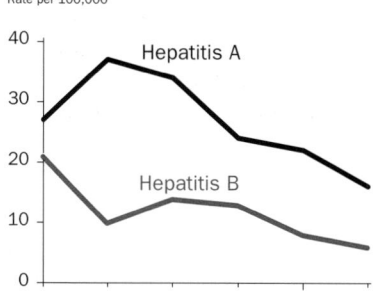

Sources: Inserm U444, RNSP.

Hepatitis B

Hepatitis B virus (HBV) is transmitted via blood, sexual intercourse and saliva: it is responsible for acute, sometimes fatal infections (fulminant forms), and serious long-term complications if the patient becomes a chronic carrier.

The incidence of infection by HBV in France has decreased over the last 15 years, probably as a result of the prevention of HIV transmission. In 1996, it was estimated at about 3,000 new cases (6 per 100,000) for symptomatic acute infections (which, in those over 5 years old, account for approximately 30 to 50% of all new acute infections); in 1991, the estimated incidence was about 10,000 cases (21 per 100,000) (figure 32). Newly acquired infections have the following characteristics: two thirds occur in men, 90% of whom are 20 years or older; the infection is acquired via intravenous drug use in 20% of cases, via sexual transmission in 35%, and via needle exposure in 15%; no risk factor is identified in about 30% of cases. Infection by HBV can give rise to fatal fulminant hepatitis, particularly if associated with infection by hepatitis D virus; in 1993, it was estimated that 15 cases of fulminant hepatitis had been caused by HBV in France.

5 to 10% of infected patients over the age of 5 become chronic carriers of the virus. Approximately 30% of chronic infections progress to cirrhosis, and the latter progresses to cancer of the liver in 30 to 50% of cases after 10 years. Available surveys of prevalence in France have been used to assess the prevalence of chronic carriers of HBV per at-risk group (table 38).

Table 38 **Prevalence of HBs antigen in various French populations, 1990-1995**
(number of cases per 10,000)

	Number of cases per 10,000
Women with NH insurance, Centre region (1991)	10
Pregnant women born in France (1992)	15
New blood donors (1996)	16
Autologous blood donors (1995)	25
New blood donors (1991)	28
Men with NH insurance, Centre region (1991)	30
Women with STD (1990)	200
Pregnant women born outside France (1992)	256
Men with STD (1990)	510
HIV+ patients (1991-1994)	690

Source: RNSP.

Thus, it has been estimated that about 100,000 persons in France are chronic carriers of the virus. Hence, they are potential sources of infection for others and are themselves liable to the long term complications of the infection. This pool of chronic infection is fed each year by about 1,000 new cases of chronic infection, minus the deaths attributable to HBV as a result of chronic diseases of the liver and evaluated at about 1,000 annually. Thus, the pool of those with chronic HBV infection will remain constant unless an extensive programme of vaccination is undertaken to prevent new infections.

Hepatitis C

Transmitted mainly *via* blood, the insidious spread of hepatitis C virus (HCV) over the last few decades accompanied the rapid development of blood transfusion; it was then introduced among the population of intravenous drug users and "exploded" and has now become the "prototype" of viruses transmitted in a hospital setting. For the past few years, chronic infection by HCV has become a prime public health concern in terms of both morbidity and cost to society.

Its prevalence among the general population (positive results in third generation serologic tests, ELISA and RIBA) was estimated in 1994 on the basis of 2 separate surveys carried out:
– among a random sample of contributors to the national insurance scheme who volunteered for a health checkup in 4 regions,
– among a random sample of all women who had terminated a pregnancy in the Île-de-France and Provence-Alpes-Côte-d'Azur regions.

The results from the 2 surveys indicated that about 1% were anti-HCV-positive. In the survey carried out among national insurance contributors (involving men and women aged 18 to 60 years), the crude prevalence of anti-HCV-positivity was 1.2%: when corrected for the age and sex distribution of the reference population, and after taking sample structure into account, the prevalence was estimated to be 1.1% (95%-confidence interval: 0.75-1.34). Eighty per cent of those who were anti-HCV-positive were carriers of the virus (RNA of HCV). However, there were inter-regional variations in the prevalence: Centre 0.8%, Île-de-France 0.9%, Lorraine 1.0% and Provence-Alpes-Côte-d'Azur 1.7%. Moreover, prevalence increased with age, especially in women. Among autotransfusion candidates who were not selected because of risk factors, there was a regular increase in prevalence with age, with maximum prevalence after the age of 70. A comparison of prevalence data led to a suggested estimate of 500,000 to 650,000 for the anti-HCV-positive population in 1994: of these, approximately 75% are unaware of their serologic status.

The importance of HCV infection in terms of public health relies on its progression to a more chronic form and the development of serious hepatic lesions over the long term. Given the known natural history of the disease, about 80% of cases will progress to a more chronic form and about 30% of subjects with chronic hepatitis C will develop cirrhosis: among the latter, the incidence of cancer of the liver is 30 to 50% within 10 years. According to this model, the incidence of chronic complications of HCV infection will be very high and very adversely affect morbidity, mortality and the medical care system. The interaction between chronic infection (more than 60% of carriers were unaware of their status in 1997) and alcohol consumption worsens the prognosis considerably and, in France, this fact will have to be taken into consideration in the strategy adopted for secondary and tertiary prevention. However, up until now, insufficient data are available on which to base accurate measurements of the infection's actual impact on public health or to make any reasonable projection, since many uncertainties remain concerning its natural history and the long term efficacy of treatments.

Treatments were initially limited in their efficacy but newer therapies are more effective, particularly if instigated early, and powerful screening tests are now available: this has led to the recommendation that active screening for HCV infection should be carried out among present or former drug addicts and persons who received transfusions before 1992. At the same time, reference centres associated with "town-hospital" networks have been set up to deal with the predictable increased load of screening activities and therapeutic management. All of these arrangements need to be evaluated.

There is no accurate information concerning the current incidence of new infections by HCV (seroconversion). Nevertheless, an estimate of the incidence of seroconversion is of major strategic value since only by knowing its incidence can the spread of HCV infection be appreciated. While transmission *via* transfusion is under control, there is still a considerable but unascertained amount of transmission among intravenous drug users, and the question of persistent nosocomial transmission still remains open to debate. In France, an estimate has been made of the incidence of infection among known blood donors, seroconversion being detected when an anti-HCV-positive blood donation was noted after a previously negative donation. Over the period 1994 to 1996, the incidence was 2.7 per 100,000 person-years. Extrapolated to the general population aged 20 to 64, the number of new HCV infections would be about 1,000 per year over the period 1994-1996 at the very least since, obviously, the risk among known blood donors is an under-estimate of the real situation.

Data derived from an analysis of the seroconversion noted among known blood donors give some indication as to persisting modes of transmission. In decreasing order of frequency, the risk factors identified among blood donors who seroconverted between 2 donations were : intravenous drug use (25%), endoscopy, all forms combined (20%), minor surgery (10%), sexual partners (8%) and professional exposure (5%). No risk factor could be detected for 32% of the seroconversions. These figures highlight two persistent routes of contamination: intravenous drug use (25%) and nosocomial exposure (30%).

This analysis of present epidemiology shows that HCV infection has to be regarded as a major public health problem, given the size of the population affected, the prognosis for HCV infection and its future social cost, and the persistent, appreciable level of transmission among intravenous drug users, in spite of current policy aimed at reducing risks, especially the nosocomial risk. Faced with this observation, it is essential that surveillance, evaluation of the screening programme and current management, and monitoring of persisting modes of transmission should all be stepped up. Further clinical research and epidemiological research into the natural history of the disease must be carried out.

Hepatitis G

Hepatitis G virus is related to HCV and they share a common ancestor. The virus was discovered in 1995 and is transmitted by blood, and possibly also by sexual intercourse. Although it can induce hepatic cytolysis during contamination in man, there are no indications so far that it is implicated in chronic liver disease. To date, the most impartial scientific and public health finding is that hepatitis G virus is "a virus in search of a disease".

Emergent and re-emergent infections

This idea was conceived in the United States at the beginning of the 1990s and widely adopted on an international scale – indeed, one department of the World Health Organisation now bears its name. Up until the end of the 1980s, there was an unprecedented decline in the morbidity and mortality due to infectious diseases not only in developed countries but also in many countries of the southern hemisphere, thanks to advances made in hygiene and vaccination, and the discovery and widespread utilisation of antibiotics. The onset of AIDS (the very prototype of an emergent disease), the development of resistance to antibiotics, the outbreak of epidemics widely publicised in the media (Ebola virus, Hantaviruses, *Escherichia coli* O157:H7, etc.), the discovery of new infective agents (hepatitis C virus, etc.), and also the resurgence of infections once thought to have been controlled by modern public health programmes (tuberculosis, diphtheria and cholera in countries belonging to the former Soviet Union bloc, yellow fever in certain African countries, etc.) have all served to quickly dampen the optimism of the 1970s and 1980s. More recently, a recognition of the importance of nosocomial infections, of a iatrogenic risk of infection (Creutzfeldt-Jakob disease and growth hormone, hepatitis C, etc.), of the importance of the risk of infection from food residues (including prion or "slow" virus diseases), increasing resistance to antibiotics and the risk of pandemic influenza related to the spread of a new strain have all confirmed the idea that nothing is certain where infectious diseases are concerned and that man is persistently vulnerable to known pathogens – and even more so to new, and fortunately rare, truly emergent pathogens.

The dynamics of infection depend on the interaction between an agent (infectious microorganism), the host and the environment. Social progress has appreciably limited infectious diseases by improving the environment (housing conditions, food, sanitation, medical management, etc.) and the resistance of the host (better nutritional status, vaccination, etc.). However, changes in the host, environment and pathogens have upset certain balances, encouraging the emergence of new risks or the resurgence of former risks among population groups. Prolonged life expectancy and survival in vulnerable patients have been achieved at the expense of greater susceptibility to pathogens and to much lower doses of infection. Pathogens may evolve either spontaneously (mutation or reassortment of avian-human virus in the case of influenza), or under antibiotic selection pressure (emergence of multidrug resistance to antibiotics). Developments in technology, methods of food production, international trade, and travel and social changes (with persistent or even increased vulnerability) have also had an appreciable effect on the environment and are the root cause of many of these new risks (for example, infections derived from food).

Part two Changes in health status

The importance of emergent or re-emergent infections should not be exaggerated: in France, for example, the incidence of tuberculosis continues to decline; however, the decline has slowed down (figure 33) and is not uniform among the various social classes. The new infective risks mentioned above truly represent fresh threats to public health, either as a whole (influenza pandemic) or limited to certain groups in the population (the destitute, drug addicts, immunocompromised patients, etc.), and their control will depend on improved detection, a better understanding of the determinants, and access to medical care for the entire population.

Figure 33 **Variation in declared cases of tuberculosis in Metropolitan France, 1984-1996**

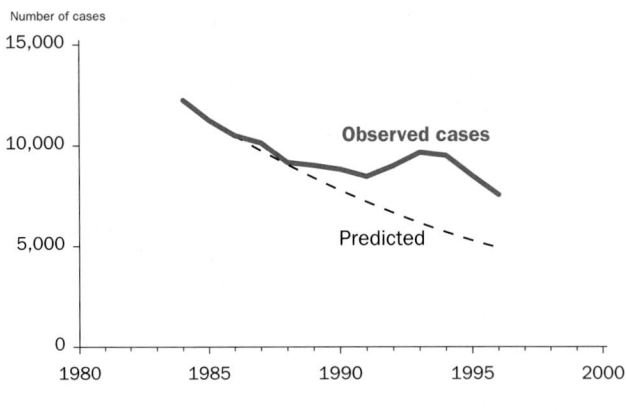

Source: RNSP.

Prion diseases: an illustration of the concept of emergent diseases

The incidence of sporadic Creutzfeldt-Jakob disease (CJD) is about 1 case per million inhabitants and has not varied over the past few decades in any of the countries where it is under surveillance, especially France. Subjects over 50 are mainly affected and the outcome is always rapidly fatal. The only clearly identified risk factors are genetic in nature. One recent European multicentre study suggested certain environmental and dietary risk factors (particularly the consumption of brains). However, assuming that these factors are the underlying cause, the risk attributable to them is very low. To this form of CJD, and apart from extremely rare familial forms, must be added iatrogenic CJD which mainly concerns children treated with certain batches of contaminated, extracted growth hormone (to date, there have been about 50 cases out of approximately 1,000 children exposed). Once again, this iatrogenic disaster illustrates the importance of applying more stringent safety standards in the utilisation of biological products of human and animal origin.

The description of a new variant of CJD (nvCJD) in 1996 in the United Kingdom, about 10 years after the start of the bovine spongiform encephalopathy (BSE) epidemic, immediately led to the fear that the bovine agent had been orally transmitted and adapted in man (consumption of products of bovine origin). Two years after the publication of reports on the first cases of nvCJD, fundamental research work on the agent responsible for nvCJD confirmed the hypothesis that the BSE prion was similar to that of nvCJD and hence that transmission from cattle to man had occurred. The most likely mode of transmission to man relies on the oral route, particularly via mechanically separated beef which has nerve tissues still attached. Modelling of the BSE epidemic in the United Kingdom indicates that of 903,000 infected cows, 729,000 as yet asymptomatic cows entered the food chain before any measures were adopted in the U.K. For the moment, 2 years of experience in the surveillance of new cases of nvCJD does not indicate that there will be any massive epidemic in man (25 cases registered to date, including 1 in France). However, it is impossible to give any estimate of its future importance.

The onset of bovine spongiform encephalopathy in the United Kingdom corresponds to the adaptation of an unusual agent transmissible to cattle, and highly effective transmission by the ingestion of meat and bone meal (MBM) of bovine origin whose chemical and heat treatment were insufficient to eliminate contamination by a prion. The origin of the BSE agent has not been clearly identified as either an agent specific to cattle recycled by the use of MBMs or as an ovine agent adapted to cattle and then recycled by MBMs. The United Kingdom epidemic was massive in scale (more than 170,000 cases) and affected several other countries, though to a much lesser extent including, more particularly, Switzerland (270 cases), Ireland (276 cases), Portugal (100 cases) and France (34 cases). The measures taken in the United Kingdom led to a huge reduction in the incidence of the disease among cattle. However, the disease continues to develop, although admittedly its incidence is low in the United Kingdom and in the herds of continental European countries, and the routes of transmission for the most recent cases (new cases involving calves born after the ban on MBMs) are poorly understood (cross contamination of MBMs during preparation, fraudulent use of MBM, vertical transmission, etc.). Moreover, it is possible that the agent responsible for BSE might be transmitted to sheep, since the ovine disease linked to the BSE agent is difficult to differentiate from scrapie in terms of clinical signs, infectious tissues and mode of transmission. This possibility might expose man to a further risk. Hence, it is of major interest to understand the epidemiology and biology of animal diseases caused by prions so that their transmission to man can be prevented.

The BSE epidemic, the onset of nvCJD, and the CJD epidemic in children treated with growth hormone illustrate the potential dangers that infections due to prions and modern technologies can pose to public health when inadequately controlled. Infections due to prions fully correspond to the concept of emergent infections discussed above.

Resistance to antibiotics

Changes in resistance to antibiotics have occurred among the majority of bacteria responsible for the most common infections: Hæmophilus influenzae, Streptococcus pneumoniæ, salmonellae, shigellae, Neisseria gonorrhoeæ, group A Streptococci, Escherichia coli. As an example, the decreased sensitivity of pneumococci to penicillin G fell over a 10-year period from 0.5% (1984) to 32% (1994), and reached almost 80% in 1996 in France. However, the prevalence of multidrug resistance in Mycobacterium tuberculosis hominis (isoniazid and rifampicin) remains stable at about 0.5%.

The development of resistance is all the more worrying since it is difficult to predict, epidemiological surveillance systems do not currently provide reliable, accurate information concerning resistance in both hospitals and the general population, and very few novel antibiotic compounds have been discovered in the last two decades.

The determinants of the spread of resistance to antibiotics are: inter-individual transmission of resistant strains and the exposure of populations to antibiotics, whether in hospitals, private medical practice or veterinary practice. Exposure of a population to antibiotics has ecological consequences that result in increased bacterial resistance to the antibiotics that have been used. In addition, it seems that the qualitative aspects of population exposure to antibiotics are at least as important as the quantitative aspects in determining such changes in resistance. Thus, the dose and length of utilisation appear to have an effect on the carriage of pneumococcus with reduced sensitivity to penicillin G (low doses and long duration). However, from an epidemiological point of view, our understanding of the relationships between the exposure of a population to antibiotics and changes in bacterial resistance is far from perfect and what applies to one bacterium/antibiotic combination cannot be extrapolated forthwith to another bacterium/antibiotic combination. Moreover, the use of antibiotics in animals – whether in the form of growth factors, medicated feed (prophylaxis) or as treatment for sick animals – induces resistance which can then be transmitted to man. This is particularly true in the case of Salmonella typhimurium which acquired a high level of multidrug resistance in animals (mainly cattle) and was then transmitted to man via contaminated foodstuffs (prime cause of salmonellosis in man, primarily children). Of these two factors (inter-individual transmission and exposure to antibiotics), the utilisation of antibiotics would seem to be the only one open to action designed to control such changes.

In order to define the most appropriate strategies to adopt in managing changes in bacterial resistance, it will be necessary to:

– arrive at a better understanding of the ecological dynamics of bacterial resistance among populations and their relationship with exposure to antibiotics, with better surveillance and pharmaco-epidemiological studies on both the utilisation of anti-infective agents and bacterial resistance;

– encourage the correct use of antibiotics by preliminary evaluation of doctors' knowledge of antibiotics and their prescribing habits and the general public's knowledge of antibiotics and its attitude towards antibiotic consumption, the development of guides for the diagnosis, treatment and prevention of community-acquired upper and lower respiratory tract infections, the development of educational strategies aimed at doctors and the general public, and the evaluation of actions implemented concerning prescribing, antibiotic consumption, and bacterial resistance.

Vaccination policy

In France, vaccination policy is drawn up by the Ministry for Health upon the advice of the "Conseil supérieur d'hygiène publique de France" (French Higher Council for Public Hygiene), and on the basis of recommendations made by the "Comité technique des vaccinations" (CTV) (Vaccination Technical Committee). This committee was set up in 1985 in response to the Ministry's request for specialised expertise in the area of vaccination, at a time of rapid changes in the vaccination schedule resulting from a combination of many factors, chief among which the following may be mentioned:

– highly ambitious, internationally established targets for controlling certain diseases (aimed at eliminating the diseases in Europe, and even eradicating them world-wide). While the ultimate hope of such objectives is the interruption of specific vaccinations, they initially require an intensification of vaccination strategies. Hence, the target of eliminating measles led to the addition of a second dose of vaccine, and corrective programmes aimed specifically at certain age groups will probably be necessary in France;

– the international epidemiological context. The diphtheria epidemic which is raging in newly independent states led to the recommendation of a reinforcing dose for those travelling to areas where diphtheria is endemic. Whether it is necessary to add further reinforcing doses in adults will ultimately be determined by means of epidemiological surveillance;

– the enormous reduction in the circulation of pathogens induced by high levels of coverage maintained over long periods, leading to alterations in the epidemiological characteristics of the disease. Thus, the very limited circulation of *Bordetella pertussis*, responsible for whooping cough, has led to the absence of any natural boost among older children and the formation of a pool of vulnerable young adults who act as a source of contamination for infants before they have completed their series of vaccinations. This phenomenon led to the resurgence of serious cases of whooping cough among very young infants in France and made it necessary to give an additional reinforcing dose to adolescents; this was made possible when new, acellular pertussis vaccines became available at the beginning of 1998. Epidemiological surveillance will indicate whether further reinforcing doses are appropriate;

– the marketing of new vaccine combinations. The recent introduction of new vaccine antigens (*Hæmophilus influenzæ* B, hepatitis B) into the vaccination schedule for infants stimulated the development of novel vaccine combinations so as to reduce the number of injections. Although the ultimate aim of basic research into mucosal immunity is to develop vaccines that can be administered orally or intranasally, *priority* will still be given in the foreseeable future to providing the medical profession with safe, effective combinations. In this connection, a hexavalent vaccine containing the hepatitis B component is expected to be put on the market in the near future and should make it easier to extend the vaccine coverage for this antigen (currently less than 50% among infants);

– the development of new vaccines. A large number of novel vaccines are presently at various stages of experimentation. For each vaccine, it will be necessary to ask whether, on the basis of not only epidemiological but also economic and sociological data, its incorporation into the vaccination schedule is relevant. A multistate application for a Product Marketing Authorisation is currently being examined for an anti-rotavirus vaccine which should become available in France at the beginning of 1999. Prime amongst those vaccines shortly expected are conjugate vaccines against pneumococcus and meningococcus C which will be effective starting from the first few months of an infant's life and will provide longer protection than currently available vaccines;

– the expansion in scientific data. Vaccines against hepatitis were marketed with the instruction that reinforcing doses be given once every 5 years. Recent studies, based on a longer follow-up period, have confirmed that the protection conferred by primary vaccination lasts at least 10 years and probably much longer – this indicates that French policy in terms of the schedule for reinforcing doses needs to be revised.

However, the implementation of vaccination policy largely exceeds mere elaboration of the schedule for vaccination since, for the policy to be applied effectively, a certain number of conditions must be met:

– the schedule must be very widely circulated and justified among health professionals and the general public. Many parties are involved in vaccination in France, making it difficult to spread the relevant information: this situation probably largely explains why vaccination coverage against measles, mumps and rubella has marked time at less than 85% among 2-year-olds. Tools such as the "Guide des vaccinations" (Vaccinations guide) and programmes promoting certain vaccinations conducted by the French Committee for Health Education are evidence of the recent efforts that have been made in this area. In this respect, it is hoped that the computerisation of doctors' offices and subsequent setting up of networks will bring about an improvement in two-way communication as far as vaccination is concerned;

– such an improvement is all the more vital since the targets of elimination/eradication require that not even a small proportion of the population be allowed to escape vaccination. Experience in Scandinavian countries and mathematical models have confirmed that the elimination of measles will demand more than 95% coverage for the two doses. In such a context, vaccination can no longer be conceived as a matter for individual choice but as a collective approach requiring full co-operation. Total compliance is all the more difficult to obtain when high levels of coverage lead to the almost complete disappearance of diseases, and fear of the side effects of vaccination can outweigh fear of the actual diseases;

– lastly, tools for monitoring and evaluating vaccination policy are essential. Basically, they must measure vaccination coverage, assess the efficacy of vaccination, monitor side effects, and deal with epidemiological surveillance.

In essence, the measurement of vaccination coverage in France relies on using information from children's 24-months health certificates. Efforts still need to be made to render vaccination coverage more reactive and exhaustive. In addition, the protective potential of vaccines must be assessed during epidemics by continuing to carry out surveys under actual conditions of use. Since vaccines are administered to healthy subjects, surveillance of their explicit side effects warrants the development of expertise aimed specifically at monitoring vaccines within the French Drug Agency. And lastly, epidemiological surveillance constitutes an essential tool for checking the impact of vaccination measures and proposing necessary adjustments to the schedule.

Such epidemiological surveillance is particularly important as an objective in interrupting the circulation of pathogens since all cases and residual infections have to be identified. Thus, enteroviruses are coming under increasing surveillance in France as part of a scheme to eradicate poliomyelitis. The targeted elimination of measles will require the same identification and laboratory confirmation of all suspected cases in view of a possible investigation. These new surveillance methods require greater co-operation between clinicians, biologists and epidemiologists who can collectively contribute to implementing vaccination policies and thereby effectively banish some of these scourges.

CHAPTER FOUR

The determinants of health status

In the present report, The High Committee on Public Health sought to tackle the determinants of health status which had not been accorded any priority in 1994. Hence, after analysing the consumption of psychoactive substances (tobacco, alcohol, narcotics), other types of individual behaviour were studied, such as driving and risky sexual practices. It was also considered necessary to introduce a section devoted to determinants linked to the physical environment and work.

Among the prime determinants of health status, the 1994 HCSP report picked out the **problems of vulnerability and social integration** from more general questions of **access to care and prevention** among disadvantaged populations.

In 1996, an HCSP working party initiated a detailed study on "increasing vulnerability in France and its effects on health" and its report was made public in February 1998[1]. In it, stress was laid not on *"extreme forms of vulnerability such as exclusion and dire poverty"* but on *"growing everyday difficulties for a large number of households which live in a situation of social instability and are left exposed by social and economic changes"*. This loss of the usual economic, social, family, etc. forms of security might affect about 20% of the population living in France. The degradation of an individual's economic situation can lead to persistent unemployment, a stream of unsteady jobs, deterioration in living conditions... and may be accompanied by a loss of self-esteem, giving rise to mental anguish which undermines good health.

Hence, in addition to the differences in health status that can be detected among the various socioprofessional categories, part of

---

1. *"La progression de la précarité en France et ses effets sur la santé"* (Increasing vulnerability in France and its effects on health), HCSP report by a working party presided over by J.-D. Rainhorn, February 1998. Rennes: Ed. ENSP, 1998, 368 p.

the population is also suffering from the specific effect of increasing social and economic vulnerability.

Thus, the number of those seeking work for more than one year rose from 846,000 in 1992 to 1,089,000 in 1996, the number of those on the minimum unemployment benefit (RMI) increased from 575,000 in 1992 to 904,000 in 1996, and the total of those receiving minimum social benefits from 2,830,000 to 3,163,000 [2].

In addition to general measures to bring about integration and social cohesion designed to prevent increasing vulnerability among the population, the working party insisted on measures that would improve access for the destitute to social and medical services, as targeted in the 1994 HCSP report.

In fact, it is estimated that, in 1996, 16% of the entire population was not covered by any supplementary system of social protection and that neither did three quarters of those concerned have any free medical assistance or exemption from payment of the "ticket modérateur" (patient's contribution towards the cost of medical treatment). This means that several million people with low incomes have only limited access to treatment, particularly dental and ophthalmological care. It should be remembered that the average rate of reimbursement by national health insurance for all medical acts and goods was the same in 1995 (74%) as fifteen years earlier, whereas it has remained at over 90% in Germany and the United Kingdom. These financial difficulties are compounded by complex administrative procedures which leave patients ignorant of their rights, unevenly applied regulations, and obvious psychological barriers. Thus, the Government's March 1998 announcement of guaranteed access to care for all, as part of the programme for preventing and fighting against exclusion, should help to achieve progress towards the target stated in the 1994 report of the HCSP.

One part of the reform, included in the law of 29 July 1998, is designed to materially improve the situation of the destitute by running regional programmes for access to prevention and care, and by reaffirming the social mission of hospitals. Beyond this, the reform sets out to create universal sickness coverage, to guarantee supplementary protection for the most destitute, and to institute exemption from advance payments.

---

2. *"Données sur la situation sanitaire et sociale en France"* (Data relating to health and the social situation in France), Ministry of Employment and Solidarity, SESI, Paris: La Documentation française, 1998.

Determinants linked to individual behaviour and the social environment

In its 1994 report, *Health in France*, the High Committee on Public Health underlined the importance of tackling avoidable premature mortality. Of the 60,000 annual deaths regarded as avoidable, it noted that 40,000 were linked to lifestyle, especially:
– deaths due to lung cancer between the ages of 25 to 64, related to smoking,
– deaths due to cancer of the upper airways and digestive tract between the ages of 25 to 64, related to smoking and alcohol consumption,
– deaths due to alcoholism between the ages of 15 to 64,
– deaths due to road accidents between the ages of 5 to 64, related to reckless behaviour.

Naturally, the High Committee on Public Health recommended that determined policies be conducted in the fight against alcoholism, smoking and road accidents. It accorded a special place to combating drug addiction and preventing HIV infection and sexually transmitted diseases.

It would therefore seem to be useful to draw up a balance sheet with dual objectives: on the one hand, for each topic emphasised by the HCSP, it must be seen whether the targets it set in terms of indicators are being attained and the measures undertaken must be identified; on the other hand, it may be necessary to discuss potential changes in the specific scope of each topic, especially in conceptual terms.

The main determinants related to individual behaviour and the social environment are analysed in the following pages: alcohol consumption, smoking habits, drug addiction, dangerous driving, and risky sexual behaviour.

Alcohol consumption

In its 1994 report, *Health in France*, the High Committee on Public Health set itself three objectives to be pursued up until the year 2000 in the fight against excessive alcohol consumption and dependency on alcohol:
– to reduce the average consumption of pure alcohol by 20% among people over 15,
– to reduce harmful behaviour and its impact on health and society,

Part two   Changes in health status

– to reduce regional disparities so as to bring consumption in all regions to the level noted in regions with the lowest consumption.

Reducing the average consumption of pure alcohol among adults

Although the average consumption of pure alcohol per person over 15 is constantly declining, it will be difficult to achieve the consumption target set for the year 2000, *i.e.* 11.3 litres.

Alcohol consumption in France has continually fallen since the middle of the 1960s.

Average consumption per person 15 years and over dropped from 22.3 litres in 1970 to 20.6 litres in 1980 and to 16.6 litres in 1990. In 1996, decreases had brought the average consumption down to 15.6 litres (figure 1).

Over the last two years, the annual decline in consumption has only been 0.6%, which is obviously insufficient for the target to be reached.

Wine still accounts for two thirds of the total consumption of pure alcohol; the consumption of "appellation contrôlée" (guaranteed quality) or superior quality wines has remained steady or even increased.

The fall in consumption is actually not uniform among the various sections of the population and masks very contrasting situations.

Figure 1   **Average alcohol consumption by people 15 and over**

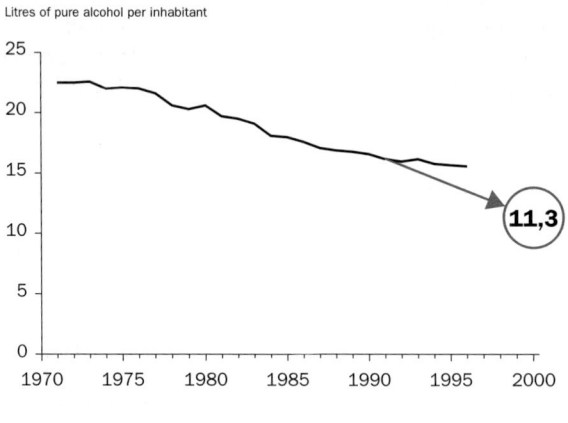

Source: Insee.

A change in behaviour: new drinking habits among the young

After a slight shift in alcohol consumption among the young between 1984 and 1991, consumption increased in 1994 and 1995 (table 1).

The determinants of health status

Table 1 **Percentage variation in alcohol consumption among the young from 1991 to 1995**
(as a percentage)

	1991	1994	1995
Regular consumption	7	4	5
Occasional consumption	40	43	60
Non drinkers	53	53	35

Source: CFES.

In 1995, 65% of the young aged 12 to 18 stated that they drank alcohol compared with 47% in 1991. Comparisons of consumption over the last ten years show that adolescents are not drinking more than they used to, but that there are fewer non-drinkers among 13-14-year-olds and 15-16-year-olds.

The increase in the number of young drinkers includes girls as well as boys.

The young are abandoning wine as the daily accompaniment to meals, switching instead to so-called "social" drinking involving "top-notch" wines. Throughout France, beer and strong spirits are the favourite drinks of young people. The consumption of strong spirits doubled between 1991 and 1995, and during those four years, the proportion of young drinkers of strong spirits shot up from 25 to 47%.

The heavy drinking patterns that lead to increased alcoholism among the young differ specifically from those in adults inasmuch as consumption is intense and intermittent, primarily at weekends, and is sometimes combined with the taking of illegal narcotics and psychotropic drugs.

Reducing harmful heavy drinking patterns and their effects on health and society

The direct consequences of excessive alcohol consumption on health can be tracked by means of deaths from main causes, alcoholism, alcoholic psychosis and cirrhosis and, to a certain extent, cancer of the upper airways.

Having recalled the limits of these indicators of mortality (cirrhosis not exclusively alcohol-related; accidents and suicides partially linked to alcohol, etc.), the High Committee on Public Health recommended that changes in these indicators should be followed up over time so that the long-term effects of excessive drinking on health could be monitored.

While for all causes combined, the mortality rates due to alcoholism for both men and women (alcoholic psychosis and cirrhosis) have plunged by almost 40% in 15 years, it should be noted that this decline has slowed since 1992: this was confirmed in 1996 (figure 2).

Figure 2 **Deaths due to alcoholism (alcoholic psychosis and cirrhosis)**
(comparative mortality rates smoothed over 3-year periods)

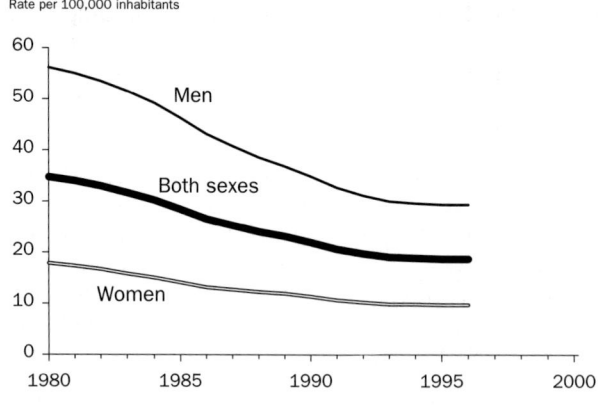

Source: Inserm SC8.

In addition, an increase has recently been observed among women in cancer of the upper airways, also related to the rise in smoking (see the chapter *Indicators of health status, "Cancer"*).

Reducing regional disparities so as to bring consumption in all regions to the level noted in regions with the lowest consumption

Analysis of the 1993/94 and 1995/96 adult health Barometers and the 1996 nutritional health Barometer confirms that the geographical distribution of global alcohol consumption and its breakdown into "wine drinkers" and "beer drinkers" no longer correspond to the traditional north-south divide. Regional disparities appear to have dwindled recently as far as wine consumption is concerned and high average consumptions of beer and strong spirits are now found scattered throughout France. In contrast, the highest percentage of beer drinkers is evidently still in the north-east of the country.

During the last four years, the overall average regional alcohol consumption has apparently not dropped to match that in regions with the lowest alcohol consumption.

Measures for combating the risk of detrimental alcohol consumption in France

During the last ten years, new factors have been introduced into the area of public health concerning alcohol consumption.

One factor relates to behaviour regarding numerous psychoactive substances, including alcohol, which could be tackled by a common approach. Another factor is the concept which has emerged of moderate alcohol consumption being "beneficial to health".

The risk related to alcohol, addictive behaviour, and reckless conduct

Up until now, all public policies directed at the consumption of potentially harmful substances have primarily focussed on the nature of the substance itself. Public policies aimed at alcohol and alcoholism can therefore be identified in the same way as those targeting tobacco and smoking, and illegal narcotics and drug addiction.

As recalled in a recent report by Prof. B. Roques[3], neurobiological and pharmacological studies have shown that all these substances act on one or more mediators, causing behavioural changes among consumers and often identical clinical signs. From a scientific standpoint, it is logical to group the different types of behaviour together under the general title of behaviour relating to psychoactive substances.

There are three basic types of behaviour: these are respectively related to normal use, abuse, and dependence.

Regardless of the substance involved, dependent behaviour has gradually been identified and has opened up the notion of addictive conduct as defined since 1990.

The following is the definition of addiction: the process by which behaviour that can elicit pleasure and also eliminate or attenuate internal malaise is expressed in a manner characterised by the repeated impossibility of controlling such behaviour, and its continuation in spite of an awareness of the negative consequences.

By itself, addictive behaviour is liable to be harmful but, in addition, it is structurally linked to other types of comportment that are potentially injurious to health: living on the fringe of society, delinquency, extravagant conduct, etc. All such types of behaviour must be grouped together and qualified as wanton, going beyond the simple framework of merely addictive behaviour.

Moderate alcohol consumption and health

It has repeatedly been shown that drinkers with a declared consumption equivalent to 1 to 2 glasses of wine per day have a lower risk of ischaemic heart disease than non drinkers – and this in many countries which have different cultural habits. This seems to indicate that a causal relationship might be involved and could be working to the advantage of the French health situation to a certain extent. Popularised sometimes as the "French paradox", this idea must obviously be handled carefully in terms of public health, but it fits in perfectly with the distinction made earlier

---

3. *"Problèmes posés par la dangerosité des 'drogues'"* (Problems raised by dangerous narcotics). Report by Prof. B. Roques to the Junior Minister for Health, May 1998.

between normal behaviour and behaviour related to abuse and even dependency.

Policies put into practice in the last five years

In 1994, the High Committee on Public Health recommended:
– putting into practice a policy for preventing heavy drinking that leads to increased alcoholism,
– developing all means and structures for assisting those with alcohol problems,
– developing actions in specialised settings,
– drawing up and implementing regional programmes,
– increasing the number of people with specialised training in alcoholism.

Moreover, in its 1996 European charter on alcohol consumption, the WHO recommended that extensive programmes be devised to fight alcoholism in member States. The programmes must accurately define their targets and indicators of results, and must monitor the progress achieved so that it can be updated following evaluation. The European department of the WHO has proposed that the strategy should encompass legislation, trading, prices, access to alcohol, and advertising.

All the evidence suggests that the public authorities have not, over the course of the last five years, defined any comprehensive plan for combating alcoholism.

Besides the standard French denial of alcoholism and the sizeable contribution made by "alcohol income" to the national economy, the lack of any defined policy probably results from the practical difficulty of using the concept of addiction. Nowadays, this global concept actually seems more suited to defining a policy of prevention than organising the management of behaviour related to abuse and dependency.

According to the report by Prof. Ph.-J. Parquet[4], messages aimed at prevention would be easier to put across if the idea of behaviour were used to replace that of the substance: the messages would have to make everyone understand that each type of at-risk behaviour can have a deleterious effect on health.

This concept becomes less effective when a system of management has to be contrived. Can generalised health care units be envisaged that will admit, for example, young drug addicts hooked on heroin and those who drink excessive amounts of strong spirits, adult men who are exclusively heavy drinkers and young women who are taking multiple drugs and smoking heavily, without any attempt at streaming them? The development of this type

---

4. Parquet Ph.-J., *"Pour une politique de prévention en matière de comportements de consommation de substances psychoactives"* (Promoting a preventive policy towards the consumption of psychoactive substances), Vanves, Éd. CFES, 1997, 107 p.

of structure is only conceivable as an experimental set-up with a strict assessment process, possibly restricted to certain sections of the population (*e.g.* management of addictive behaviour in adolescents...).

Obviously, the absence of any national overall plan for fighting alcoholism has not hindered the implementation of health measures aimed at both prevention and care.

The policy of prevention

Both the demand and supply of alcohol have been equally targeted by prevention policy.

Regulations concerning the supply of alcohol are essentially designed to control drinking establishments, to ensure the protection of minors, and to supervise advertising for alcoholic beverages. To this end, the law of 10 January 1991 (the so-called "loi Evin") restricted the conditions for advertising the "substance alcohol".

Since 1991, not all the decrees stating measures for enforcement of the law have been published. The content of the "alcohol" section of the law has gradually been watered down by successive amendments (advertising by billposting in manufacturing areas, regulations for refreshment stalls at sports stadia, etc.).

Is this context propitious for evaluating the "loi Evin" as statutorily launched on 24 March 1997? The overall decrease in the number of litres of pure alcohol drunk by the average French individual during a period in which the law failed to be applied could lead to the conclusion that there is no need to legislate in this sphere. It has to be remembered that alcoholism is still a major public health problem in France and that, in spite of its imperfections and limitations, the "loi Evin" is highly symbolic, channelling the emergence of a new public health culture concerning at-risk behaviour related to alcohol.

Prevention in terms of the demand for alcohol has basically relied on nation-wide programmes with the messages: "un verre, ça va... trois verres, bonjour les dégâts!" (one glass is OK... but after three, watch out!), "Tu t'es vu quand t'as bu?" (Have you seen yourself when you're drunk?), and "l'alcool, où en êtes-vous?" (How far have you gone with alcohol?). It can be seen that such programmes have gradually brought in the idea that citizens should be aware of their responsibilities. But is this concept tailored to all sections of the public, especially its youngest members?

At the local level, these programmes have been taken over by community structures: results have been variable since the resources available in each region differ. But on the whole, prevention suffers from numerous points of discord among regulatory provisions that encourage consumption on the one hand, and preventive messages that extoll moderation on the other. The promotion of moderate consumption using health-based arguments does not help to clarify the area of communication.

Patient management

In the past few years, no re-definition has been given of the management of patients with alcohol problems. However, intra-hospital liaison teams specialising in alcoholism have been set up (circular DH/EO4/96 of 10 September 1996) and the promotion of networking has been encouraged (circular DGS/SP3 of 19 November 1996).

The task of trained alcoholism teams is to assist in the management of problems throughout health care establishments, in terms of both the alcoholic patients and the medical care teams.

Teams have the following objectives:
– to refuse the usual denial of problems and be able to tackle them with the patients,
– to help patients express their request for help and management,
– to guide patients towards the alcoholism team during the hospitalisation period and the "follow-up structures" at the time of discharge.
This new direction taken by hospital policy has yet to be evaluated.

Taking into account the course defined by the HCSP, the National Health Directorate tried to respond to the need for early, total management of those who abuse alcohol or are alcohol-dependent, by encouraging networking among the parties involved. The policy relies on three main lines of action:
– providing general practitioners with information and raising their level of awareness,
– supporting the setting up of specialised alcoholism teams for liaison purposes,
– training and forming a network of the various participants. In 1996 and 1997, 6 million francs were committed for this action so as to sustain the work carried out in 20 French regions which had selected alcohol as the primary health determinant at regional health congresses (8 of these regions launched their own programme).

Smoking

At the present time, three million people die world-wide every year as a result of smoking. The number of deaths attributed to smoking in the European Union is estimated at 548,000 per year. Forecasts for 2010-2020 run at 10 million deaths per year over the whole world, including two thirds in developing countries. In particular, a marked progression is expected in female deaths. 10 to 30 years from now, mortality due to lung cancer in women will doubtless exceed the toll due to breast cancer.

In 1990, it was estimated that 60,000 deaths were tobacco-related in France, including 5,000 female deaths. Based on current trends in consumption, forecasts of smoking-related mortality for the year 2025 are pessimistic (160,000 deaths, including 50,000 in women, *i.e.* a 10 times multiplication).

The HCSP regards the battle against smoking as a major stake in public health, requiring the instigation of a determined policy. In 1994, four targets were set for the year 2000:
- to reduce tobacco sales by 30%,
- to reduce the proportion of regular smokers in the adult population by 25%,
- to reduce the proportions of regular and occasional smokers in the 12-18 year age group by 35%,
- to reduce the proportion of women who continue to smoke when pregnant.

Reducing tobacco sales by 30%

Tobacco sales are falling every year in France. Between 1991 and 1997, they fell from 103,870 tons to 92,300 tons, *i.e.* an 11.2% decrease in 6 years. However, the most recent data have shown an upturn in sales (+ 1.1% for cigarettes and + 4% for cigars in the first six months of 1998).

Since 1992, the average consumption per person over 15 decreased by approximately 10%, total tobacco consumption dropping from 6.1 to 5.5 g/d, the amount of tobacco smoked in the form of cigarettes declining from 5.7 to 5.0 g/d (figure 3).

If the target set by the HCSP for the year 2000 is to be achieved, an annual drop of 5% will have to be recorded between 1996 and 2000. Over the last three years, the average annual drop has been about 3%.

However, although cigarette sales have fallen by 14.5% since 1991, purchases of bulk tobacco have risen by 43%. In fact, increasing the price of cigarettes has certainly encouraged a shift in consumption towards bulk tobacco, especially the roll-your-own variety. However, because of its small share of the tobacco market (4.8% of tobacco sales in 1990, 7.4% in 1996), purchases of the cheaper product fail to compensate for the disenchantment with cigarettes.

Compared to other European countries, tobacco consumption in France is average (table 2).

An analysis of European statistics confirms that there is a link between cigarette consumption and their sales price. Greece, for

Part two Changes in health status

The smoking habits of adolescents are linked to those of their entourage: friends exert a major influence in encouraging the start as well as the cessation of smoking.

Parents also play a decisive role in their children's smoking habits when they smoke themselves or have a more or less permissive attitude towards smoking.

There is also a link between the socioprofessional category of the parents and smoking among adolescents. The higher the social category, the more pocket money the young have at their disposal, and the more likely they are to smoke.

On an international scale, young French people were not the most numerous in declaring that they had already tried smoking. On the other hand, a WHO survey conducted in 21 countries ranked France in 7th place in terms of the proportion of regular smokers among 11-year-olds, 3rd among 13-year-olds and 9th among 15-year-olds.

Reducing the proportion of women who continue to smoke when pregnant

The perinatal health surveys carried out in 1981 and 1995 showed that the percentage of women who smoked during pregnancy had risen.

The proportion of women smoking at least one cigarette per day before becoming pregnant increased from 27% in 1981 to 39% in 1995, and the same change was noted in women who smoked during the third trimester of their pregnancy (from 15% to 25%, i.e. currently one woman in four).

Policies implemented 1994 and 1998

In 1994, the High Committee on Public Health recommended:
– increasing the tobacco tax by 15% per year, for an overall increase in retail price of 70% by the year 2000,
– organising a specific action aimed at health professionals so as to set an example,
– making drug-based and other techniques aimed at helping people to stop smoking more readily available,
– integrating the fight against smoking in school programmes and intensifying health education in schools with the aim of delaying the age at which both boys and girls begin smoking,
– helping pregnant women to avoid smoking by offering them appropriate support.

Since 1994, the fight against smoking has to be seen from an international perspective. In fact, major cigarette manufacturers are multinational corporations with a world-wide strategy.

1996 was marked in the United States by negotiations between the three biggest tobacco manufacturers and the Attorney Generals of certain States of the Union.

The agreement, which doubtless will finally not be validated at the federal level, basically made provision to relinquish the right to institute any proceedings against manufacturers in the future for reasons of health in return for the payment of 368 thousand million dollars over 25 years.

In any case, the current situation among manufacturers in the United States and many European countries is spurring them to become much more aggressive in marketing to developing countries.

In Europe, a proposal for a directive prohibiting the advertising of tobacco products has been under discussion for almost 10 years. For economic reasons, many countries have, in fact, opposed the ban on advertising relating to smoking.

On 4 December 1997, the European Council of Ministers for Health reached an agreement to ban direct and indirect advertising for smoking and the sponsoring of cultural and sporting activities by tobacco manufacturers.

The interval allowed before the directive must be adopted as national law is three years from the time publication in the "Journal Officiel" with, however, a longer interval for the printed press (4 years) and sponsoring (5 years). A special dispensation has been granted for Formula 1 racing, eight years being allowed before the directive is adopted as national law without, however, overstepping 1 October 2006. The text sets out a dispensation to allow States which, like France, already have more stringent regulations, to preserve their present arrangements.

It should also be noted that the ban on tobacco advertising will not apply to publications which are printed and issued in third countries and not primarily intended for the European Community market.

Actions for the prevention of smoking that are being conducted in France are aimed at both sides of the problem, demand as well as supply.

Action aimed at the supply of products

The first regulation introduced for tobacco products dates back to 9 July 1976. The "loi Veil" limited advertising for cigarettes, particularly on billboards, and authorised it in the printed press under certain conditions. It also prohibited the distribution of free tobacco. Additionally, Article 4 of the law specifically stated that no objects in common use other than those directly serving for the consumption of tobacco or tobacco products could be offered, handed out, or distributed if they carry the trademark, name or advertising logo of a tobacco product.

However, while the "loi Veil" had the merit of existing and being the first regulation in the matter, difficulties were encountered in its implementation since it failed to form part of an overall disposition and was relatively little applied by the tribunals.

The "loi Evin" of 10 January 1991 came into effect on 1 January 1993, amending and reinforcing the 1976 legislation. It prohibits all forms of tobacco advertising, whether direct or indirect. Since the law came into force, the tobacco advertising surveillance agency has noted a 95% reduction in illegal advertising expenditure.

Moreover, for the first time, the "loi Evin" gave the public authorities the possibility of freely increasing taxes, which represent over 70% of the sales price, placing tobacco outside price indexes and leading to a 77% increase in the price of a packet of cigarettes in 5 years (figure 7).

Smoking in public places has also been prohibited since November 1993. This legislation is designed to combat passive smoking and also to limit the effects of imitation which encourage the use of tobacco.

In December 1995, six Regional Health Surveillance Centres published a survey concerning evaluation of the application of legis-

Figure 7 **Average daily consumption of tobacco per person aged 15 and over compared with changes in its relative cost**

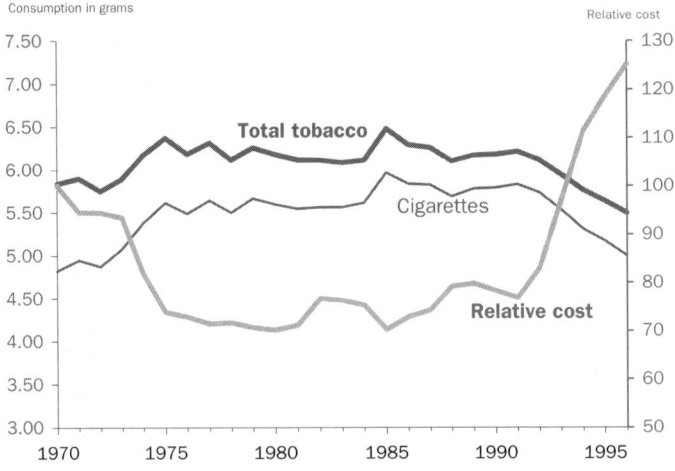

SEITA convention: 1 cigarette = 1 cigar = 1 cigarillo = 1 gram of tobacco.

Sources: Insee, Seita.

lation relating to the protection of non smokers[5]. The survey revealed that one firm in two had not made any special arrangements, and that the regulations were not observed within the French educational system (45% of children, 40% of supervisors and 20% of teachers had been seen with a cigarette inside school grounds).

Although the ban on tobacco advertising has been observed since January 1993, other forms of promotion have developed, for example private parties subsidised by tobacco manufacturers with free distribution of cigarettes.

In terms of education and health training, the State and CNAMTS devote about 20 to 25 million francs per year to prevention programmes on television and actions in the field, but there does not appear to be any real co-ordination between the various parties involved.

Action aimed at demand

It is important to remember that the consequences of smoking on health status are not all irreversible and that stopping smoking is a good idea at any age. The speed at which harmful effects lessen varies with the risk in question (relatively rapidly for the vascular risk, and much more slowly for cancer and especially respiratory failure). Accordingly, it is essential to actively promote the cessation of smoking.

The earlier an individual takes up smoking, the greater the risk of developing a smoking-related disease. The prime aim must therefore be to try and influence the young, but to do this, adults must be urged to stop smoking so as not to set a bad example.

Dependence on tobacco results from pharmacological, social and psychological factors. The pharmaceutical industry has developed certain methods to assist in nicotine withdrawal. Nicotine-based drugs allow the smoker to undergo a gradual suppression of the conditioned reflex (smoking) without experiencing the unpleasant symptoms of withdrawal.

The efficacy of the various methods (chewing gum, patches, etc.) depends on the subject's degree of motivation and dependence. The use of combinations produces considerably better results than those obtained by each separate method. Psychological counselling helps to make the methods even more effective.

Methods not based on drugs have also been developed for aiding in withdrawal. However, it is difficult to determine just how effec-

---

5. ORS Bourgogne, Centre, Champagne-Ardenne, Limousin, Haute-Normandie, Poitou-Charentes, *"Évaluation de l'application de la législation relative à la protection des non-fumeurs"* (Assessment of the application of legislation concerning the protection of non smokers), 1995, 59 p.

tive they are. Repeated advice from the subject's attending physician, although not in itself a withdrawal method, is certainly an effective technique in the fight against smoking.

Nevertheless, two types of difficulty are encountered. Firstly, general practitioners still too often lack credibility since a considerable percentage are smokers themselves. And secondly, general practitioners are still inadequately trained with regards to tobacco withdrawal.

Lastly, the impact of methods which solely affect those who spontaneously seek help in quitting the smoking habit is still very small, even though the methods are effective.

Drug addiction

In the fight against drug addiction, the High Committee on Public Health recommended focussing action on the following three targets in 1994:
– to reduce heroin consumption without increasing the consumption of cocaine or cocaine derivatives,
– to reduce the risk of health problems in drug addicts, especially new cases of AIDS and hepatitis,
– to facilitate the social integration of drug addicts.

Reducing heroin consumption without increasing the consumption of cocaine or cocaine derivatives

Given the illegal status of narcotics, available statistics concerning their consumption are scattered and piecemeal.

Changes in the consumption of illicit drugs in France have been estimated on the basis of some existing sources of data. Basically, the data are derived from the national file of those found guilty of infraction of the narcotics legislation ("Office central de la répression du trafic illicite des stupéfiants", OCRTIS (French Narcotics Bureau)), statistics from services responsible for the management and monitoring of drug addicts, and surveys carried out for CFES health Barometers.

Indictments for narcotics use or use and dealing

Between 1980 and 1995, indictments for narcotics use or use and dealing in narcotics climbed from 10,187 to 62,325 (figure 8).

Between 1992 and 1995, the increase was over 25%: in 1995 alone, a 19% rise was noted.

This augmentation concerned all types of narcotics, but indictments were mainly for the use of cannabis. The number of indictments for simple heroin use or use and dealing in heroin remained steady in 1992 and 1993, and even rose slightly in 1994 and 1995 (figure 9).

Figure 8 **Interpellations for simple narcotics use or use and dealing in narcotics, as a function of the product involved, 1980-1995**

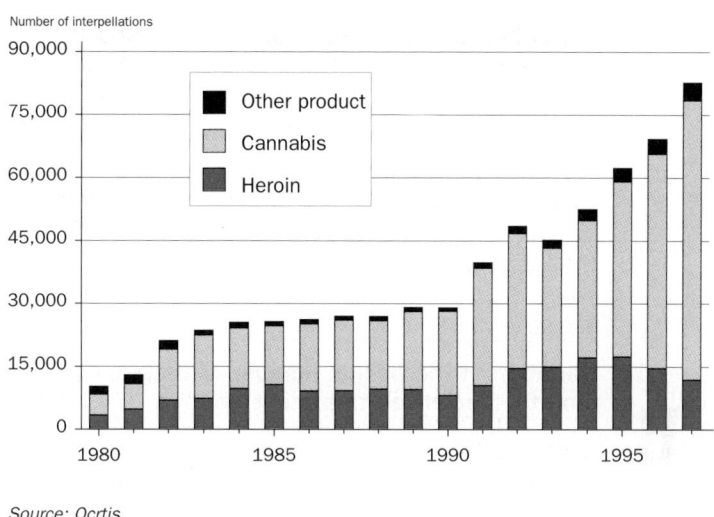

Source: Ocrtis.

Figure 9 **Interpellations for simple narcotics use or use and dealing in narcotics, 1972-1997**

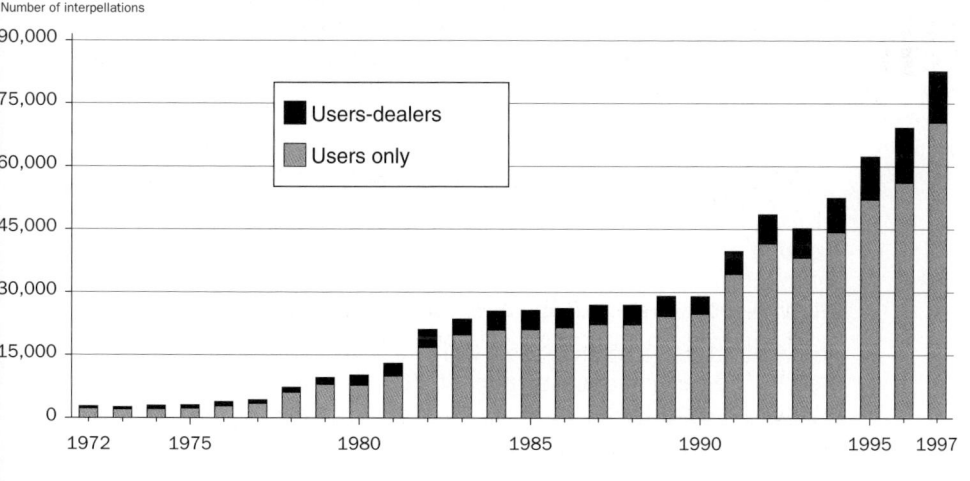

Source: Ocrtis.

In part, the increases were due to greater efficiency on the part of the police in fighting drug addiction. However, this explanation must not be allowed to hide the fact that there has been an increase in illegal drug use in France, and one of its effects can be measured from the extent to which drug addicts seek admission to health and social care centres.

Admission of drug addicts to health and social care centres

The number of drug addicts who sought help in specialised centres rose from 31,762 in 1990 to 64,738 in 1995, *i.e.* an increase of over 100% (figure 10). In 1995 alone, a progression of more than 22% was recorded.

Figure 10 **Variation in the annual number of drug addicts seeking admission to specialised treatment centres**

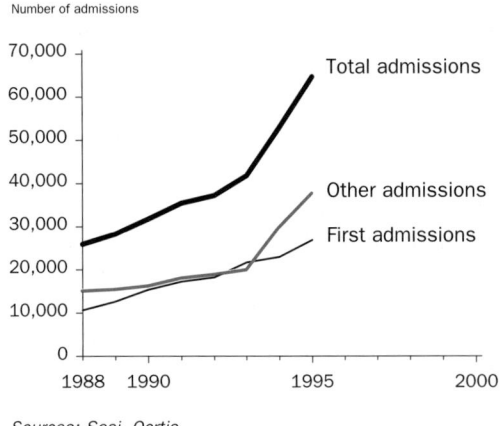

Sources: Sesi, Ocrtis.

An analysis of admissions to the health and social care system also gives a measure of changes in the types of drug used among the population of those admitted. In November of every year, SESI conducts a survey in all establishments belonging to the health and medico-social system to find out how often drug addicts seek help.

In 1995, 10,871 admissions were related to the utilisation of heroin, *i.e.* an increase of almost 70% in 5 years for this substance (figure 11).

Surveys of behaviour among various populations
Consumption among adults

According to the 1995/96 Health Barometer survey among adults, there was a slight increase in the proportion of persons who admitted having taken drugs during their lifetime relative to 1992 (12%

Figure 11 **Variation in the number of heroin users admitted to health and social care structures for the management of heroin addicts**

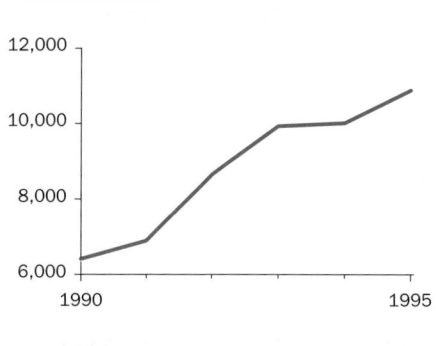

Sources: Sesi, Ocrtis.

in 1992 compared with 16% in 1995), although the proportion of persons who stated that they had taken a drug during the previous 12 months showed no change (4% in 1992 and 1995).

Cannabis was still the most frequently taken product and the proportion who admitted taking it during their lifetime increased between 1992 and 1995 (15% in 1995 *versus* 11% in 1992).

Drug consumption over the course of a lifetime is both sex- and age-related. More men admitted to drug-taking behaviour – 21% had taken a drug at least once, compared with 11% of women.

Drug-taking is also more prevalent among the young: 32% among those aged 18-24, and only 1.5% among those in the 60-75 age bracket.

In addition, the number of students who admit to taking drugs during their lifetime has been increasing since 1992: 24% in 1995 *versus* 17.5% in 1992.

One survey was carried out in 1995 in army selection centres (DCSSA) among young men aged 18 to 22 and investigated drug consumption by means of an interview with a doctor and analyses of urine. The results showed that:
– cannabis is still the product most often taken: 19% of those interviewed stated that they had taken cannabis within the previous three months and it was detected in 16% of urine specimens,
– cocaine and heroin use were admitted by 0.7% and 0.6% of subjects respectively: tests were positive in fewer than 0.2% of cases.

Experimenting with drug consumption is also linked to a subject's socioprofessional category. More students and those in management and intermediate professions have experimented with a drug during their lifetime than members of other socioprofessional groups.

Consumption among adolescents

The most recent figures concerning drug consumption among adolescents date from 1993. One adolescent in 7 at school had already tried a drug, while this proportion was 22% among the young seeking employment (half of whom admitted taking drugs at least 10 times).

The national survey of adolescents conducted by M. Choquet and S. Ledoux (INSERM) in 1994[6] showed that, among 11-19-year-olds, 85% had never taken drugs, 6% had experimented once or twice, 3% had taken drugs between three and nine times and 5% at least ten times.

The drug most often taken by adolescents is hashish (12%) compared with cocaine (1.1%) and heroin (0.9%).

Among those who take hashish or marijuana, almost 40% do so regularly (at least 10 times), whereas regular users account for only 20% in the case of other products.

More boys take drugs (18%) than girls (12%). Some differences are age-based: 6% of boys and 3% of girls aged 11 to 13 have taken an illicit drug, while the corresponding figures are 39% and 22% among boys and girls aged 18 and over.

Among psychotropic drugs, illegal products account for 15% of consumption (of which 1/8th relates to hashish and 1/100th to so-called "hard" drugs). The survey confirmed that excessive consumption occurred among the children of those in management, children at secondary school, and the young whose parents had separated.

Young people who frequent cafés and night clubs, or who hang about in the streets have a four times greater risk of becoming drug addicts than others of the same age.

A new product: ecstasy

A far greater diversity has been noted in the products used by drug addicts in the past few years. In fact, while heroin consumption is tending to shrink, drug users – especially the youngest drug users – have turned to other products and have sometimes become addicted to several drugs.

Introduced in France in the 1980s, ecstasy is a synthetic product which was initially presented as a psychotropic agent with stimulant and aphrodisiac properties.

---

6. Choquet M., Ledoux S., *Adolescents*, Paris, Éd. INSERM, 1994, 346 p.

At first, it was confined to a small number of persons in groups of "swingers", then spread in the 1990s to a much broader, younger public and is no longer used as a "happiness pill" but as a stimulant and pep pill.

The growth in ecstasy consumption was accompanied by the introduction of certain styles of music (House, Techno, etc.) and notably by "rave-parties" (gatherings of sometimes very large numbers of young people and adolescents).

Indictments for the use of ecstasy have shot up from 32 in 1990 to 1,122 in 1995.

The most recent studies (1998 INSERM collective expert appraisal[7]) have demonstrated the toxicity of ecstasy, and the fact that it sometimes even leads to the subject's death.

In outline, ecstasy has several effects: euphoria, empathy, a feeling of bodily well-being... Its harmful effects are complex and generally appear after several doses have been taken. Primarily, they consist of anxiety disorders and depressive states accompanied by insomnia. The user may also experience blood pressure disorders, palpitations, tremors, nausea, amnesia and confusion.

The pilot research study on ecstasy conducted in 1997 by the "Observatoire français des drogues et des toxicomanies" (OFDT) (French Surveillance Centre for Narcotics, Addictions, and Substance Abuse) showed that the population concerned was inclined to be young and male. 70% of users are considered to be between the ages of 18 and 25. However, unlike the case with cannabis, few adolescents use ecstasy: 4% in 1995.

Of the subjects included in the sample, 45% were salaried employees, 22% were students and 20% practised a liberal or artistic profession: most were unmarried. While the population was mainly male, it should still be noted that female users of ecstasy outnumbered female users of cannabis by 2 to 1.

Where prevention is concerned, and in spite of the inaccurate data, it would seem that user awareness of the toxicity of ecstasy is highly inadequate. Most ecstasy users do not consider themselves as drug addicts.

Those who take ecstasy do not often seek help in specialised centres, and those who do are either addicted to multiple drugs and regard their consumption of ecstasy as "trivial", or they have encountered physical or psychological complications.

In conclusion, the HCSP target of trying to reduce heroin consumption does not appear to have been achieved and, given the intro-

---

7. *"Ecstasy: des données biologiques et cliniques aux contextes d'usage"* (Ecstasy: laboratory and clinical data under normal conditions of use), Paris, INSERM, Expertises collectives, 1998.

Reducing the risk of health problems in drug addicts

duction of new drugs and new methods of consumption, strategies for prevention will have to be defined.

There are no accurate figures for the mortality rate among drug addicts. However, it is estimated that a thousand drug addicts died of AIDS in 1995. As for deaths due to overdose, OCRTIS data indicate that there was an increase up until 1992 (500 cases), followed by a plateau up until 1995[8]. During the latter period, between 200 and 250 additional deaths annually could be singled out in which drug use was specified as an associated cause of death.

The number of new AIDS cases among intravenous drug users dropped dramatically in the 2nd quarter of 1996 following a period of stabilisation between 1992 and 1995. From 1996 to 1997, it decreased by 55%. Obviously, information is very fragmented as far as the spread of HIV among drug addicts is concerned. Data collected in Aquitaine reveal a continuing decrease in the annual number of intravenous drug users who have discovered that they are seropositive since the start of the 1990s *(see the chapter Indicators of health status, "Transmissible diseases")*.

Policies adopted between 1994 and 1998

In 1994, the High Committee on Public Health recommended:
– reinforcing prevention and the management of vulnerable young people before they reach adolescence,
– reducing recourse to injection by developing a substitution policy,
– reducing the time between the first injection and the first request for care,
– promoting health education among drug addicts by using contact centres, and developing syringe-exchange programmes,
– improving the socio-economic integration of drug addicts and reinforcing inner-city policies,
– improving the mental health of this population by increasing the capacity of specialised addiction centres.
As part of the policy of risk reduction, various measures were promoted so as to avoid health problems arising.

Substitution

The governmental plan of 21 September 1993 set up new procedures for the management of drug addicts, with substitution as one of its guidelines.

A circular dated 9 November 1993 suggested developing the practice of substitution which had so far been under-utilised.

---

8. Observatoire français des drogues et des toxicomanies (French Surveillance Centre for Narcotics, Addictions, and Substance Abuse), *"Drogues et toxicomanies"* (Narcotics, Addictions, and Substance Abuse), 1996, 127 p.

Within the scope of the methadone programme, any community or hospital medico-social institution which could guarantee global management of drug addicts was allowed to request up to 50 places for use in methadone substitution therapy.

Current substitution policy relies on two types of product: methadone and Subutex® (buprenorphine); the scope for use of the latter was defined by the Advisory Committee for Substitution Therapy created on 7 March 1994.

Methadone may be prescribed by all centres specialising in the care of drug addicts. General practitioners have been involved in prescribing such therapy once the first phase of monitoring has been completed in a specialised centre.

In 1996, specialised care centres which prescribe methadone for drug addicts were set up in ten new departments and it is estimated that in a 3-year period about 84 centres were authorised to offer substitution therapy. 4,000 persons were monitored in these centres in 1996, and an additional 600 treated with methadone were monitored in private practice.

Subutex® has had a marketing authorisation since 31 July 1995 and has been available from retail pharmacies since February 1996.

This drug can be prescribed by any attending physician after a medical examination as part of overall therapeutic management for patients who are heavily opiate-dependent and already being monitored in private practice. In September 1996, 19,000 persons were being treated with Subutex®.

Departmental committees were set up on 31 March 1995 in order to provide follow-up on the substitution policy. The aim of such committees is to contribute to organisation of the prescribing of substitution drugs by installing networks covering specialised care centres for drug addicts, doctors and pharmacists, and also to advise health professionals and see that new substitution drugs are used correctly.

Revival of the treatment injunction

The treatment injunction – so called ever since a ministerial circular in 1984 – was defined in Article L 628-1 of the Public Health Code and appeared to have been definitively abandoned at the start of the 1980s.

In spite of two 1987 circulars encouraging the implementation of the treatment injunction, it was not until the beginning of the 1990s that it was finally incorporated into a comprehensive arrangement (governmental anti-drug plan of 21 September 1993).

An interministerial circular of 28 April 1995 concerning the harmonisation of practices relating to the treatment injunction made provision for reinforcement of the treatment injunction procedure, an alternative to legal proceedings against users of narcotics. Before resorting to the treatment injunction procedure, prior judicial proceedings must have taken place.

The treatment injunction represents an alternative to legal proceedings and hence cannot be envisaged unless it is suitable for the drug addict concerned. Hence, the 1995 circular only makes provision for resorting to this procedure in the case of users of narcotics such as heroin or cocaine, or for those who take massive amounts of cannabis or in combination with other products. Provision is also made to resort to the treatment injunction when the user is a minor taking heavy doses or is addicted to several drugs.

The DDASS (Departmental Division for Health and Social Affairs) is responsible for monitoring the treatment, either by means of the medical health inspector, or by a specific team.

Ministry of Justice data concerning treatment injunctions since 1992 show that the will to revive the handing down of treatment injunctions resulted in an actual increase in such injunctions (table 4). In effect, the number handed down rose from 6,149 in 1993 to 8,630 in 1995.

However, these figures hide considerable inter-regional dissimilarities which are particularly apparent when the number of treatment injunctions are compared with the amount of jurisdictional activity concerning narcotics. Some jurisdictions still seem reluctant to hand down treatment injunctions.

Table 4 **Number of injunctions and medico-social follow-ups of drug addicts in 1993, 1994 and 1995**

	1993	1994	1995
Number of injunctions handed down	6,149	7,678	8,630
Number of persons who actually had medico-social monitoring	4,064	5,760	6,072

Source: DGS, SED.

Promoting preventive actions

Preventive measures must be taken very early so as to preclude all types of at-risk behaviour in children and adolescents who are not on drugs.

This means initially putting greater effort into educating the young by giving suitable training to all those who play a role in teaching.

The determinants of health status

A certain amount of training has been given in this way to teachers, instructors, personnel working in reception centres, members of the police force, etc. Direct actions among the young have also been developed, mainly by giving them immediate, anonymous access to the information that they seek.

Youth information centres, centres for documentation and information in junior and senior secondary schools, local missions, social centres, etc. keep a certain amount of information on drug addiction at the disposal of young people. Educational steps have also been taken using cultural and sporting events to get the message across and, by keeping track of the young, making it possible to intervene at an earlier stage.

Prevention also means avoiding the transition from occasional use to abuse and then dependence.

For this reason, 2,000 social environment committees have been set up in junior and senior secondary schools so that the Head of school is surrounded by a permanent network of interlinking skills, created inside and outside the institution and devoted to finding ways of handling young people showing signs of drug abuse.

The network of local missions and "permanences d'accueil, d'information et d'orientation" (PAIO) (24-hour reception, information and guidance facilities) receive almost 1,300,000 young people per year, including 200,000 who have major problems.

Within the context of the risk reduction policy, the development of places for making contact with drug addicts has resulted specifically in the creation of "boutiques": 32 have so far been opened.

These places receive the farthest fringe of non-detoxified drug addicts, most of whom are excluded from specialised care arrangements for drug addicts. They provide an opportunity for opening up a dialogue, listening and informing drug addicts, and also for eating, washing and receiving nursing attention.

The intention of the circular of 11 January 1995 concerning continuation of the plan to fight drug addiction was to explore all possible means for reaching out to the far-fringe drug users who had not sought treatment. Teams were set up to operate on the streets and tailor reception and suitable services to the situation of such addicts.

The policy of risk reduction also includes making syringes available to drug addicts. The development of Steribox continues: since September 1994, approximately 6.5 million preventive kits have been sold. Monthly sales are showing a big increase: 192,000 kits sold per month in 1997 compared with 162,000 in 1995.

Similarly, 86 syringe-exchange programmes have been set up, and 148 automatic dispensers, exchangers-dispensers or recovery units for syringes have been installed.

Management

The 1993 government plan made sweeping changes in the system of management for drug addicts.

The plan now operates along four main lines: substitution, development of contact centres for drug addicts, setting up networks involving drug addicts, private practice and hospitals, and specialised arrangements for the medical care of drug addicts.

Networks involving drug addicts/private practice/hospitals are designed to improve the management of drug addicts. The 50 networks have become a means of co-operating between all those involved, and they ensure liaison and treatment continuity at the different sites of patient management.

Hospital management has developed along five central themes:
– continuing mobilisation of hospital departments with respect to their tasks in detoxification,
– greater emphasis on medical consultations,
– setting up of teams for liaison and medical care of drug addicts,
– strengthening of certain hospital departments involved in the management of drug users and obliged to deal with crisis situations,
– training of hospital personnel.

There are two types of specialised care arrangements: specialised medical care centres for outpatients, and medical care centres with lodging facilities. Specialised medical care centres for outpatients are responsible for global management that includes monitoring drug addicts in medical, psychological, social and educational terms.

One of the objectives of the 1993 government plan was to double the capacity of centres with lodging facilities for the management of drug addicts. From 720 places in 1993, such centres now have 1,395 places. The centres have not only increased their lodging capacity but have also diversified and now offer structures better suited to the requirements of drug addicts.

Thus, side by side with treatment centres having collective accommodation (former post-detoxification lodgings), there also exist sections with networks of families providing care and lodging for drug addicts who, after withdrawal treatment or substitution therapy, wish to break with their usual environment, and sections of relay-treatment apartments.

The determinants of health status

Road accidents

In 1994, the target set by the High Committee on Public Health was to halve the number of injuries and deaths on the roads by the year 2000.

Changes in mortality

Road deaths dropped from 10,285 in 1990 to 8,412 in 1995, i.e. a decrease of about 18%. At the same time, there was a decline in the number of injured and in the gravity of the accidents (table 5). 20% of those killed on the roads were young people aged 18 to 24.

Accidents tend to be less serious as the area where they occur becomes more urbanised. But whatever the size of the built-up area, accidents are always more serious at night than during the day. Two thirds of all accidents occur at night and they cause slightly more than half of all road deaths.

Fatal accidents mostly occur on main and secondary roads which are more dangerous than motorways.

International comparisons do not show France in a particularly good light and it ranks far behind the United Kingdom and Holland.

Table 5 **Accidents involving bodily harm and death**

	Accidents with bodily harm	Killed	Injured
1990	162,573	10,289	225,860
1991	148,890	9,617	205,968
1992	143,362	9,083	198,104
1993	137,500	9,052	189,020
1994	132,726	8,533	180,832
1995	132,949	8,412	181,403

Source: Interministerial Road Safety Surveillance Agency.

Changes in behaviour

Four types of responsibility are involved in causing accidents, and obviously more than one may be to blame:
- the responsibility of the user in about 90% of cases,
- the responsibility of the infrastructure in about 50% of cases,
- the responsibility of the vehicle in 20% of cases,
- general driving conditions in 20% of cases.

The human factor is to blame in two ways in 90% of accidents, i.e. due to undesirable behaviour and/or being unfit to drive.

Undesirable behaviour

Drinking alcohol, driving fast and not wearing a seat belt are important factors involved in respectively 48%, 30% and 24% of fatal accidents (according to "Réagir" surveys carried out after serious accidents). In about 20% of accidents, drivers are unfit to drive, basically because they are overtired.

Speed

Since 1995, the speed limit on motorways and in built-up areas has tended to decrease whereas it is slightly increasing on main roads and in villages.

The number of speeding offences showed a sharp drop in 1993, then rose slightly in 1994-1995, stabilising at about 1,150,000 (table 6).

Table 6 **Number of speeding offences**

	Number of offences
1985	933,253
1990	1,153,539
1991	1,259,590
1992	1,273,184
1993	1,107,112
1994	1,145,778
1995	1,165,347

Source: Interministerial Road Safety Surveillance Agency.

Blood alcohol concentration

Since 15 September 1995, a blood alcohol level of between 0.5 and 0.8 g/l constitutes a class 4 minor offence; above this limit, it becomes an indictable offence entailing two years of imprisonment, a 30,000 F fine and the loss of 6 driving licence points.

In the case of accidents involving bodily injury, the blood alcohol concentration of not only the driver but also of all passengers able to drive is routinely screened. In fact, current case law tends to bring proceedings against passengers who, though not themselves under the influence of alcohol, knowingly allowed an individual with a blood alcohol concentration higher than the permitted level to drive.

Between 1995 and 1996, the number of positive alcohol screening tests following accidents involving material damage and bodily injury decreased by 3.9% and 4.7% respectively (1996 annual statement of the Road Safety Surveillance Agency).

However, the number of positive results from spot checks carried out during preventive controls increased during the same period. The lower level of alcohol permitted in blood and a more than

6-fold increase in the number of spot checks between 1985 and 1995 might very well account for this increase.

Wearing seat belts

Although failure to wear a seat belt does not cause accidents, it does adversely affect the outcome of accidents.

Surveys carried out by the "Institut national de recherche sur les transports et leur sécurité" (INRETS) (National Institute for Research on Transport and Safety) among a sample of drivers revealed that they generally felt that wearing or not wearing a seat belt ought to be a matter of personal choice since it did not put anyone else in danger.

Wearing a seat belt became mandatory for those in the front of a vehicle in 1975. Since the decree of 27 December 1991, seat belts are mandatory for the driver and passengers in both the front and the back of the vehicle. In addition, children under ten years old must be transported in an approved strap system.

The proportion of those wearing seat belts has been steadily increasing since 1986, including in built-up areas (table 7).

Table 7 **Percentage of persons wearing seat belts in private vehicles** (as a percentage)

	1986	1989	1992	1995
Motorways	76	90	94	96
Secondary roads	72	85	90	93
Roads in small towns	65	82	87	90
Large cities				
Paris	33	48	53	71
Province	37	56	62	72

Source: Interministerial Road Safety Surveillance Agency.

It was decided in 1994 that not wearing a seat belt would mean the loss of one driving licence point and this appears to have been an effective means of dissuasion.

However, although the recorded number of offences decreased between 1993 and 1995, it increased in 1996 without any conclusive reversal of the trend.

At the end of 1996, a preventive campaign was conducted on radio and television and in the printed press by "Prévention routière" (Road Safety) and the French Federation of insurance companies on the topic of driver responsibility.

Fatigue and inattention

It is difficult to isolate fatigue as a factor in accidents since the latter can just as well result from lack of sleep or a sleep disorder, too much time spent at the wheel before the accident, or the taking of medication.

Fatigue is held to have been the sole, primary or secondary cause of an accident in 20% of cases when the persons involved have alleged that they were physically tired and/or had been driving for longer than two hours. When the driver is dead, only the length of time at the wheel can be considered.

Information programmes have been run throughout France, urging drivers to stop every two hours.

Actions and regulations since 1994

Since 1994, many regulations and preventive measures have been introduced, most of which are designed to directly affect the behaviour of motorists.

On 17 December 1993, the Interministerial Road Safety Committee decided to reinforce road safety along the following 4 lines: by expanding prevention, improving training, making the system of dissuasion more effective, and ensuring the safety of vehicles and the infrastructure.

Safety, training, and prevention

To increase vehicle safety, a decree of 5 July 1994 made it mandatory to carry out a technical control once every two years for private cars over four years old.

As for training, youngsters under 16 years of age must now obtain a road safety certificate to be able to drive a moped (decree of 1 July 1996). Since the decree of 5 May 1994, drivers and passengers alike must also wear a crash helmet.

In terms of prevention, the State and three major groups of insurance companies signed an agreement on 15 November 1994 whereby the insurance companies undertook to devote 0.5% of insurance premiums for civil liability to preventive measures for a period of three years.

At the Community level, the European Commission recently put forward a strategy designed to reduce the number of road accident victims in Europe by 18,000 by the year 2001. The four main topics tackled were:
− road infrastructure and environment,
− vehicles and vehicle accessories,
− information, programmes, raising public awareness,
− education and road safety training.

Legislation and regulations

In terms of legislation, a new code of criminal law came into effect in 1994 making it possible to indict, as an offence imperilling others, a certain number of different types of behaviour usually punished by a fine.

The offence defined in the new Article 223-1 of the code of criminal law consists of directly exposing others to the immediate risk of death or injuries such as to cause mutilation or permanent disablement by the overtly deliberate violation of a specific obligation for safety or caution enjoined by the law or regulations.

This legal article, whose conditions of application were defined in the circular of 24 June 1994, makes it possible to indict certain types of driving behaviour, particularly drunken driving and exceeding the speed limit which have not caused any damage but which could have done so in certain circumstances.

In terms of regulations, most were aimed at the principle causes of road accidents defined above.

Thus, the decree of 5 May 1994 prescribes that young drivers must observe a speed limit below the ordinary legal speed limit for two years after obtaining their driving licence. Young drivers must restrict their speed to 80 km/h on main roads and 110 km/h on motorways.

In the area of road safety, the High Committee on Public Health proposed updating legislative and statutory arrangements in the fight against drunken driving. A decree of 11 July 1994 instituted a class 4 fine for drivers with a blood alcohol level equal to or greater than 0.7 g/l. This measure was complemented by a decree of 15 September 1995 which lowered the maximum permissible blood alcohol concentration from 0.7 to 0.5 g/l. Anyone found driving with a blood alcohol level equal to or greater than 0.8 g/l is guilty of an indictable offence. Hence, the reduction of the legal blood alcohol level while driving from 0.8 g/l in 1983 to 0.7 g/l in July 1994 and 0.5 g/l in August 1995 met with the recommendations of the HCSP.

A law of 26 February 1996 stipulated that these sanctions also applied to those accompanying learner-drivers.

Government bill concerning various road safety measures

While there has been a real reduction in the number of accidents involving bodily harm between 1994 and 1996, the targets set by the HCSP in 1994 are still far from being attained.

In 1996, France recorded almost 125,500 accidents involving bodily harm, with 170,117 injured and just over 8,000 dead. 20% of those killed on the roads were young people between the ages of 18 and 24 years.

Part two   Changes in health status

The decrease in the number of persons killed is tending to become smaller, while the accidents are becoming increasingly serious.

Faced with this observation, the French Cabinet adopted a government bill involving various road safety measures on 18 February 1998. Thus, the government set the target of halving the number of those killed in road accidents within five years.

To this purpose, five provisions were made:
– the first concerns those who have held a driving licence for less than two years who commit an offence punished by the loss of at least 4 points on their licence. From now on, these offenders will have to undergo a training programme designed to raise awareness of the causes and consequences of road accidents (law of 10 July 1989 on the driving licence with points);
– the second provision concerns driving instruction and provides for a mandatory written contract to be drawn up between driving schools and their clients, and requires additional sureties from those who teach in, or run, such schools. Prefectorial powers will, moreover, be reinforced so that the prefects may suspend certification or teaching licences if criminal proceedings are involved;
– thirdly, the government bill provides for the institution of pecuniary liability on the part of the holder of the registration certificate in cases of speeding, and failing to stop at red lights and stop signs;
– in addition, Article 5 of the government bill provides for repeated speeding at more than 50 km/h over the limit to be made an indictable offence. This indictable offence is punished by 6 months of imprisonment and a fine of 50,000 F and will also entail the loss of 6 points from the offender's driving licence;
– lastly, provision is made so that drivers involved in fatal accidents are automatically screened for narcotics.
This provision will allow the judge to take into account the results obtained in deciding on the punishment.

Risky sexual behaviour

During the last ten years, the development of social sciences in the area of sexuality – partly due to the gravity of HIV infection – has led to a new understanding of the sexual behaviour of the French.

New approaches to French sexual behaviour

Transition from the idea of sexual risk to that of sexuality risk

Obviously, the notion of risk in the field of sexuality concerns not only the probability of contracting a disease (the most serious being HIV infection) as a result of sexual intercourse, but also the likelihood of starting an unwanted pregnancy...

Here, the idea of zero risk is equivalent to a complete absence of sexual intercourse or the strict application of methods of protection. The teachings of social science put this idea in perspective, making it necessary to analyse risky behaviour in terms of each individual's specific sociocultural, economic, political and affective context.

As in other areas, the study of risk in terms of sexuality questions the theory that human behaviour is rational and picks out separate economic, affective and cognitive, and sociological approaches to risk.

The economic conception of desired utility can be applied to preventive behaviour. An individual will adopt risk-free behaviour if the satisfaction anticipated from such behaviour outweighs the risk. One example would be the acceptance of unprotected intercourse by a prostitute: if the need for money is greater than the fear of contracting a disease, the individual will then throw caution to the winds.

According to workers who develop cognitive theories, an individual arrives at a decision after having decoded, analysed and organised a multitude of pieces of information in order of their priority. This theoretical approach postulates that psychological variables predominate in the choices made by an individual. Where sexuality is concerned, theory places amorous feelings as an important factor in the taking of risks.

From the sociologists' viewpoint, individual behaviour is largely conditioned by constraints imposed by social structures. Hence, the social environment plays a major role in helping to shape the behaviour of any given individual.

Taking these sexuality risks into account, N. Bajos showed that during the 1990s, whether behaviour designed to provide sexual protection was adopted depended on the socio-economic, political, cultural and ideological milieux in which individuals moved, the characteristics of their surrounding social circles, their social representations in terms of sexuality, their social and sexual ambitions and, lastly, the nature of their affective and sexual relationships. Thus, an individual's perception of whether his/her behaviour is risky seems to be a complex variable which does not necessarily play a key role in inciting preventive behaviour.

AIDS: the only sexual behaviour-related risk to receive media attention

At the start of the 1980s, infection with HIV burst onto the scene of sexuality and profoundly affected methods and indicators used in analysing French sexual behaviour.

While surveys paid more attention to sexual technique, the AIDS era obliged research workers to devote greater attention to behaviour that helped spread contamination and to incorporate far more epidemiological items into their surveys (number of different partners over a given period, utilisation of condoms, etc.).

Similarly, funds earmarked for research into French sexual behaviour have greatly increased and made it possible to acquire further knowledge useful in developing campaigns for prevention.

Changes in sexual behaviour

While AIDS extensively contributed to the blossoming of surveys into sexual behaviour, the surveys themselves were often fragmentary and oriented towards populations identified as being at-risk. Only the 1992 survey, "Analyse des comportements sexuels des français" (ACSF) (Analysis of French sexual behaviour) conducted among 20,000 persons in France[9] measured changes which had occurred in this domain since 1972, when the last global survey known as the "Simon survey" was carried out. The other surveys (KABP 1994, survey of sexuality among adolescents, survey of sexual behaviour in the French West Indies and Guyana, surveys among the homosexual community) provided a degree of enlightenment which, though limited, was of fundamental importance in defining specific strategies.

The ACSF survey: changes in sexual behaviour between 1972 and 1992

The age at which young people have their first sexual experience has remained stable since the 1970s: 17 years for men, 18 years for women. The length of their sexually active life has grown longer, particularly among women; 50% of married women over 50 were sexually active in 1972, and 80% of women with a partner aged 50 to 69 in 1992.

Between 1972 and 1992, there was no increase in the average number of sexual partners during a man's lifetime (12 in 1972 and 1992), nor in the frequency of sexual intercourse. The frequency of homosexual encounters has remained stable: approximately 4% of men state that they have homosexual relationships.

Between 1972 and 1992, women had more sexual partners (3.2 in 1992 compared with 1.8 in 1972). There has been a sharp decline in prostitution. Women are finding a greater degree of satisfaction in their sexual life, whereas it has remained unchanged for men.

Different strata of the population exhibit various types of behaviour imprinted by social, economic and cultural factors, particularly in terms of the age of the first sexual experience (earlier in lower

---

9. Spira A., Bajos N., ACSF Group, *"Les comportements sexuels en France"* (Sexual behaviour in France), 1993, Paris, La Documentation française, Rapports officiels, 352 p.

social classes). However, the diversity in types of behaviour cannot be interpreted as merely being due to differences in social milieu, and sexual lifestyles have to be considered as independent of social characteristics.

The 1994 KABP survey

In order to ascertain how much French people knew about HIV infection and how it affected their practices, so-called KABP national surveys were carried out in 1992 and 1994 by the "Agence nationale de recherche sur le sida" (ANRS) (National AIDS Research Agency) and the "direction générale de la Santé" (DGS) (National Health Directorate) among random samples of the French population aged 18 to 69.

Between 1992 and 1994, respondents developed a better understanding of the modes of transmission of HIV, and the entire population learned a greater degree of acceptance of persons with HIV.

As far as prevention was concerned, three main facts emerged from the 1994 survey relative to 1992:
– the general public found it more acceptable to institute routine, mandatory screening for HIV under certain circumstances;
– condom use had increased (from 22% to 27%), essentially among those under 30;
– multiple partners were less frequent (from 15% to 11%).

Survey of sexual behaviour among 15 to 18-year-olds

In 1992 and 1993, as part of an overall population survey into French sexual behaviour, A. Spira made a more detailed analysis of risky behaviour in terms of HIV among 15 to 18-year-olds living in Metropolitan France.

The survey was carried out by the BVA institute among young people attending secondary schools, training centres for apprentices, pre-professional integration programmes, and training organisations.

The following facts should be noted where prevention is concerned:
– more than half of those aged 15-18 years have sexual intercourse. At 15, more than half flirt, and barely one third have had any sexual experience, whereas at 18, three quarters have had some experience;
– 35% of boys and 24% of girls aged 15-16 claim to have already had several sexual partners, and by 18, the figures are respectively 50 and 40%;
– a condom was used during their first sexual encounter by three quarters of the young in 1994, compared with only 56% in 1989;

Part two Changes in health status

– the pregnancy rate is 3.3% among adolescent girls who have had sexual intercourse; 72% underwent an elective abortion;
– 15.4% of girls and 2.3% of boys state that they were forced into sexual acts.

Behaviour of homosexuals

The greatest changes in sexual practices have occurred among the homosexual community over the last few years, as was shown by the 1995 "Presse Gaie" survey (2,700 respondents).

It confirmed that the practice of using protective measures had been maintained at a high level, but also revealed that the unfailing use of protection was being abandoned or was difficult to maintain, primarily during occasional encounters.

Lassitude towards protective practices was evident from:
– the increase in the number of homosexuals with multiple partners. In 1991, 27% of men stated that they had had more than 10 partners during the year: this figure rose to 31% in 1993 and 34% in 1995. An increase was noted in all age groups, but especially among 16-20-year-olds, 31-35-year-olds and those over 50;
– the increased frequenting of commercial meeting places which are known to multiply the risks of contact with HIV (table 8).

Other indicators show that screening tests for HIV are requested more frequently: of those surveyed in 1993 and 1995, 48% and 65% respectively said that they performed several tests per year.

Table 8 **Percentage variation in the frequenting of meeting places** (as a percentage)

	1989	1993	1995
Public places	58	57	56
Social networks	30	31	33
Shops and stores	38	50	60
Electronic mail	37	46	43

Source: Presse Gaie.

Determinants related to work and the physical environment

The environment is a term which covers very broad areas and applies to the overall environment of the entire population as well as to environments specifically related to performing occupational tasks.

Populations directly exposed to physical, chemical or biological pollution **by virtue of their occupation** are usually exposed to much higher levels (and sometimes for far longer) than the general public is exposed to the same pollution but under very different conditions. It should be recalled that almost all the agents known to be carcinogenic in man were originally identified among populations exposed during the course of their work; asbestos may also be cited as an example, where estimates of risks corresponding to environmental levels are derived exclusively from data compiled in an occupational setting. It is currently admitted that about 5% of all deaths due to cancer in industrialised countries are work-related, *i.e.* at least 5,000 deaths every year; the figure for manual workers is at least 20%. There are other notable health problems which are either partially or wholly due to the working environment: musculoskeletal disorders (at least 30% of adult males suffer from lower back pain which is linked to working conditions to a great extent and, for the past several years, an actual epidemic of periarticular conditions has been observed developing in all countries with reliable data), impairment of hearing (related to industrial noise), reproduction disturbances, non tumoral respiratory disease, dermatological, neuropsychiatric and cardiovascular diseases, etc. In addition to physicochemical and biological pollution, it is now known that psychosocial factors associated with the organisation of work also have an effect, with repercussions on both somatic and mental health. Thus, although usually underestimated, socially discriminatory and economically unsound, occupational diseases constitute a considerable burden.

And yet it is often possible to act effectively – preventively – on the problems involved: the technical and organisational measures are frequently well recognised, French legislation theoretically provides all the means to apply the measures, and occupational medicine and a factory inspectorate can ensure their correct implementation on the spot.

Work-related activities are liable to create hazards for the general population through "passive" exposure. There are many examples: asbestos (industrial installations or asbestos clean-up operations may be close to population centres, premises con-

Part two   Changes in health status

structed with asbestos-containing materials may release asbestos during maintenance operations and affect those inside), noise, pollution of the air, water or foodstuffs by industrial sources, etc. Obviously, industry is not the only source of environmental risks for the general population – the risks may be of natural origin or linked to various human activities, such as driving cars or heating households.

A few topics of particular importance have been selected in the present chapter: atmospheric pollution concerns the general environment, while periarticular disorders and diseases caused by exposure to asbestos are primarily the result of the workplace environment.

Lastly, a report is given of recent data dealing with compensation for work-related health problems in France.

The population's general environment

Changing ideas

We all have our own personal idea of what is meant by "the environment" and it generally depends on the setting in which we live and under what conditions – ranging from individual to collective, from familial to occupational, from rural to urban, from local to planetary. To these various dimensions, some would add the notion of an environment that is not merely passively undergone but also the result of selection, thereby enlarging its scope to encompass behaviour. However, for users, the environment usually boils down to the world as they see it, in terms of physical media (air, water, soil, food, etc.), professional and personal living conditions, physical and chemical insults and biological stress.

The notion of environmental health was recently popularised by the WHO, broadening the former "hygienic" view to include positive interactions (advantages) and negative interactions (disadvantages) between health and the environment. At the same time, a less anthropocentric approach emerged with the idea of "ecology" which studies the relationships of living creatures with each other and their setting, basically in physical and biological terms.

Increasing complexity

Some of the environmental factors liable to interact with health are of natural origin, while others are associated with human development. Exposure may be acute (as in accidents, etc.), chronic (micropollution), intermittent (water, foodstuffs), or continuous and alternate (pollution in the surrounding atmosphere or inside premises). Signs of toxicity, infection or allergy may occur over the short, medium or long term.

Measures for control and prevention have been set up in industrialised countries and have lowered the biological and toxic risks linked to exposure to high doses of contaminants, other than during accidents. Above all, the present situation is characterised by chronic exposure to relatively low doses of many contaminants, making it difficult to estimate actual exposure (difficulty in measurement), to estimate the risk (effects are often weak, and populations are heterogeneous in terms of their biological reactivity), and to infer the causes of the results observed (simultaneous exposure to a multitude of interacting contaminants).

In France, there are scientific reasons why, in addition to methodological obstacles, difficulties are encountered in determining the relationship between health and the environment – little research is conducted in this area, the facilities are scattered, few laboratories have sufficient critical mass and interdisciplinary skills, and co-ordination is poor. This weakness also results from inadequate training in environmental health, which is still not well developed and organised. However, there are also structural reasons related to compartmentalisation and pronounced decentralisation of the administrations concerned and the fact that many partners are involved without any real co-ordination. This splintering of skills makes it difficult to gain access to knowledge and it hinders the mechanisms for aligning research and action.

Changes are necessary

The following five fundamental "components" must be known in order to determine the health risks related to environmental factors: the source of the pollution, the nature of the pollutants, the exposure, the dose, and the effect. The first four parameters can be found by physical, chemical and microbiological measurements and essentially they characterise the quality of the media and the potentials for exposure. This approach is certainly necessary, but often relies on a view of the environment that is too sector-based: the media (air, water, soil..., pollution (noise, waste...), and the products of "consumption" (foodstuffs, chemicals...). In part, it results from intellectual and institutional compartmentalisation, and it will have to evolve towards a more integrated, all-encompassing vision of the idea of exposure, and give greater consideration to the notions of media, and routes of input or combination of contaminants.

The health approach is the ultimate objective of health-environment research, but has been far less developed in terms of experimental work or human observation (*i.e.* epidemiology). Sometimes considered as an indicator of the quality of the environment, health can be measured at a clinical, functional level, and also at a biological level. Advances in analytical chemistry, biochemistry and molecular biology have allowed the development of biological markers, thereby taking individual susceptibility into

Part two Changes in health status

account, and providing markers for the internal dose, biologically effective dose, early response, or disease.

Thus, for the concept of environmental health to become truly operational, it is now necessary to create conditions such that specialists and cultures – still too far apart – can get together. Only a multidisciplinary approach that groups together metrologists, doctors, epidemiologists, engineers, biologists, toxicologists, and hygienists, etc. will allow us to understand as much as possible about the impact of environmental factors on human health.

From uncertainty to decision

Be this as it may, the relationships between health and the environment are, and will remain, complex. Above all, environmental health is an area that calls for decision in an uncertain situation. And yet, we must take decisions and then act. When reaching a decision in the face of uncertainty, it would be worthwhile to look more closely at new approaches which have so far been little developed in France, such as risk evaluation methodology.

The example of atmospheric pollution has been selected to illustrate this report. Obviously, other equally important areas could have been tackled, such as the pollution of tap water, but it would have meant having to present lists of facts and figures and this would have been out of place in the present report.

Atmospheric pollution

Many sources contribute to atmospheric pollution. Man is permanently exposed to micro-environments which differ widely in nature and pollutant concentration: housing, workplace, transportation, air breathed in etc. It can readily be appreciated that it is a difficult task to evaluate the effects on health related to overall atmospheric exposure of individuals if, in addition, the exposure resulting from surrounding tobacco smoke and work activities is also taken into consideration. This chapter is restricted in scope to atmospheric pollution and excludes problems linked to the ozone layer and greenhouse effect which are difficult to analyse in terms of health at the present time.

The predominance of car-related pollution

In most industrialised countries, technological advances made in the 1960s, the emission standards imposed, and the changes in energy sources in the 1970s considerably reduced the pollution resulting from industrial emissions and heating (concentrations of sulphur dioxide, SO_2, have been continuously declining over the last four decades: in Paris, for example, there has been an eightfold decrease in the annual average level since the 1950s).

Since the end of the 1970s, the number of cars on the road has grown and with it the nature of the pollution has changed. In fact, road use by private vehicles doubled in France between 1970 and 1992 while that of goods haulage rose by 70%: at the same time, rail traffic decreased by 27% and water-borne traffic by 37%. In a 25-year period, the number of private vehicles per thousand inhabitants increased from 250 to slightly over 400 in France. At the present time, there are almost 29.5 million vehicles, including approximately 24.5 million private vehicles and 5 million commercial vehicles. Accordingly, the proportion of mobile sources contributing to emissions, especially fine particles, has increased relative to fixed sources and urban pollution appears in the new guise of photo-oxidant pollution. In towns and surrounding suburbs, this situation is characterised by peaks in pollution which occur under adverse meteorological conditions and can reach high levels for several consecutive days.

There has been a radical change in the problems of atmospheric pollution since the 1970s. The local, winter peaks in pollution due to SO_2 and dust have tended to give way to summer smogs, or more complex, diffuse pollution, with a high concentration of hydrocarbons, oxides of nitrogen, oxidising compounds and very fine particles. Air pollution has also shown a more marked tendency to be regional, extending over wide distances.

At the present time, the main public health questions being asked are: What impact do current levels of atmospheric pollutants have on health? More particularly, what effects are pollutants related to car emissions having on health? And what is the impact of pollution peaks on public health? No rational decisions can be taken until at least some partial answers to these questions have been found.

Convincing, convergent results in terms of short-term effects

Much research work has been undertaken in the last few decades to back up the links between atmospheric pollution and health. Results are now available that concern a complete set of health criteria ranging from the most serious, death, to the earliest types of involvement as measured by functional or biochemical parameters. An association is consistently found between all these criteria and the levels of atmospheric pollutants, and similarly there is agreement between results that have been derived from studies conducted among various populations in very diverse economic and geographical contexts – all of which makes the overall inference as to the cause of such results quite convincing.

The studies show that even relatively low levels of pollution are linked to short-term effects on health. Daily variations in the indicators commonly measured by surveillance networks for atmospheric pollution (sulphur dioxide, SO_2; black smoke particles; nit-

rogen dioxide, NO_2; ozone, O_3) are associated with daily variations in mortality, hospital admissions for respiratory and cardiovascular problems, an exacerbation of symptoms in asthmatic patients, and a decrease in pulmonary function in children. These effects are noted at pollution levels below the exposure limits defined by air quality standards. The Aphea[10] multicentre study was carried out in 15 European cities and revealed the following for an increase of 50 µg/m³ in daily pollution levels:
– a rise of 1 to 3% in total mortality (non accidental), 4 to 5% in mortality due to respiratory causes and 1 to 4% in mortality due to cardiovascular causes;
– an augmentation in the number of daily hospital admissions: of 1 to 3% for respiratory conditions in patients 65 and over; of 1 to 8% for asthma in children; of 1 to 4% for chronic obstructive pulmonary disease.

It would be interesting to have an estimate of the potential years of life lost associated with this increase in the level of pollution but, given the study's methodology, this is unavailable.

Studies carried out among populations that are, *a priori*, sensitive (such as asthmatic patients), have shown that atmospheric pollution is a triggering factor for attacks of asthma and respiratory symptoms. For an increase of 50 µg/m³ of SO_2 or particles, an increase of between 30 and 60% is noted in respiratory symptoms, accompanied by a 4 to 8% decrease in pulmonary function. Decreases of about 2 to 4% in expiratory volume have also been detected in relation to atmospheric pollution, particularly among children who are not sick.

In general, such respiratory symptoms result from either the direct toxicity of the pollutants, or from weakened body defence mechanisms involved in allergic, viral or bacterial attack. Nevertheless, other systems are also affected by atmospheric pollution, especially the cardiovascular system. Although individual susceptibility to atmospheric pollutants is highly variable, some populations are more sensitive than others in terms of effects on health. This is particularly true for the elderly and persons suffering from chronic respiratory diseases (subjects with asthma or chronic bronchitis) or cardiovascular diseases, the variation in sensitivity depending on the pollutant considered. Children also form a sensitive population since their respiratory system is still developing and many of their activities take place outside the home.

Since pollution is now predominantly due to the transportation of goods and individuals, particularly in urban areas, vehicular traffic

---

10. Quenel P. *et al.*, "Impact sur la santé de la pollution atmosphérique en milieu urbain: synthèse des résultats de l'étude Aphea (Air pollution and health: a European approach)" (Impact of urban atmospheric pollution on health: summary of results from the Aphea study), *BEH* 1998; 2: 5-7.

has become one of the prime causes of the effects of urban pollution on the health of exposed populations [11].

Uncertainties concerning long-term effects

Over the long term (10-20 years), our knowledge is still incomplete concerning the effects of atmospheric pollution on the annual mortality rate, life expectancy and the prevalence of certain chronic diseases (chronic bronchitis, lung cancer), both in respect of experimental studies which are little suited to answering the question, or epidemiological studies requiring demanding protocols and for which it is hard to estimate subject exposure over a long study period. Nevertheless, the results suggest that there is a relationship between certain types of lung cancer and pollution due to cars, as well as a decrease in survival in cases of prolonged exposure to polluted air.

In the United States, the estimated excess risks related primarily to increases in the level of particles of about 20 to 30 $\mu g/m^3$ have been put at respectively 17% (cardiorespiratory mortality) and 26% (lung cancer). They might lead to differences in life expectancy at birth of 1 to 1.5 years between the populations of the most polluted and least polluted cities.

The magnitude of the differences and the specificity of the causes of death concerned lend weight to the theory that long-term air pollution induces chronic diseases or accelerates their development.

The public health stakes

In France, as in all industrialised countries, it is undeniable that anti-atmospheric pollution policies have contributed to an improvement in air quality over the course of the last 30 years. However, the situation in France is characterised by the size and growth in number of diesel vehicles on the road: in 1981, they represented slightly less than 9% of the total number of vehicles (private and commercial) compared with 30% in 1994. Diesel vehicles formed more than 47% of light vehicle registrations in 1994, and France is the country with the highest rate of changeover to diesel vehicles in Europe. Manufacturers are expecting the number of diesel vehicles to triple between 1980 and 2000. In addition, forecasts up until the year 2010 are anticipating a rise of 50 to 100% in the traffic on main roads and motorways, and an augmentation of about 40% in the number of cars on the road relative to 1990. Road haulage might increase by 81% by the year 2010, while rail traffic and water-borne traffic is expected to be stable

---

11. WHO, *"Véhicules à moteur et pollution atmosphérique: impact sur la santé publique et mesures d'assainissement"* (Motor vehicles and atmospheric pollution: impact on public health and clean-up measures), 1992, 256 p.

or even decline[12]. Lastly, urban and suburban traffic recorded a much higher increase than that of collective transportation. More than half of urban journeys are now made by car, and many of them are over a short distance – on average, less than 3 km in one case out of two.

Results from epidemiological studies carried out in the last ten years agree in showing that, on the whole, currently encountered urban levels of atmospheric pollutants are "very probably" a risk factor for health. The results also indicate that the upper exposure limits are not fully effective in protecting public health and, above all, that there does not appear to be a threshold below which there is no perceptible effect.

However, the question of the effects of atmospheric pollution on health often reduces to that of the impact of pollution peaks. The underlying idea is that if the consequences of the peaks were brought under control, the question of atmospheric pollution would be solved in terms of public health. Yet most epidemiological studies, such as the Erpurs[13] study in the Île-de-France region or the Aphea study in Europe, which both contributed to making the question of urban atmospheric pollution topical again in France, did not specifically study pollution peaks. They provided a general relationship between pollution levels and health risks which was established by including all of the pollution values, not only the highest observed. The media-oriented manner in which the question of the relationship between atmospheric pollution and human health is tackled on the basis of episodes limited in both time and space is a relic from the past. It is reminiscent of the 1950s and also the 1960s when high levels of pollution in cities, sometimes for several weeks at a time, led to real epidemics of morbidity and mortality. Procedures for preventing atmospheric pollution – mainly of industrial origin, at that time – relied solely on the notion of sounding an alarm. When certain thresholds had been exceeded, the public authorities implemented police measures that obliged heavy industry to use less polluting fuels, or that even directed certain installations to stop operating. It has yet to be shown that such a conception of prevention is still relevant, given that mobile sources have become the main cause of pollution.

The question of the impact of pollution peaks on health must not, therefore, overshadow the importance of background pollution on health. Although the peaks are socially perceived as "health alert" situations, they are not necessarily the predominant risk factor in terms of public health. Any interest focussing exclusively on such

---

12. Orfeuil J.-P., *"Éléments pour une prospective Transports Énergie Environnement en Europe à horizon de 20 ans"* (Prospective European Transportation, Energy and Environment 20 years from now), report by INRETS-SRETIE convention, March 1993.
13. Erpurs, *"Impact de la pollution atmosphérique urbaine sur la santé en Île-de-France, 1987-1992"* (Impact of urban atmospheric pollution on health in the Île-de-France region), ORS Île-de-France, 1995, report, 104 p.

peaks might cause neglect of preventive actions designed to reduce background levels of atmospheric pollution and might orientate preventive policies towards strategies less effective in reducing mortality and morbidity attributable to atmospheric pollution. Admittedly, atmospheric pollution is not nowadays a major public health problem in France. Nevertheless, exposure is inescapable, and there is a high proportion of vulnerable populations (those with asthma, chronic obstructive pulmonary disease, cardiovascular conditions), so that the imputable risk is appreciable. For example, in the Paris region, a 2% excess in cardiovascular mortality related to acid-particulate pollution represents between 250 and 350 deaths and 22,000 hospital admissions per year. In France, the excess risk in towns having more than 250,000 inhabitants (19.5 million persons) has been estimated at between 2 to 5% for cardiovascular mortality related to car-derived particles: this represents between 660 and 1,050 deaths per year[14].

THE "LAW CONCERNING THE AIR"

Increasing preoccupation with the effects of atmospheric pollution on health led to the adoption by the authorities on 30 December 1996 of a law concerning the air and the rational utilisation of energy. It states that *"The State and public institutions, territorial organisations and private individuals must work towards [...] a policy whose objective is to satisfy each individual's recognised right to breathe air which is not detrimental to health"*. To this end, *"The State, with the support of territorial organisations, [...] must monitor the quality of the air and its effects on health and the environment"*. Thus, since January 1997 a programme in 9 cities coordinated by the "Réseau national de santé publique" (National Public Health Network) has been studying methods of organising epidemiological surveillance, including metrological surveillance indicators of air quality and routinely collected health indicators. Any recommendations that may result from this experiment will be known at the end of 1998.

Working environment
Arriving at a better understanding of working conditions and occupational exposure

In France, little is known about the frequency and distribution of prevailing different types of working conditions and exposure to physical, chemical and biological pollutants, although several other countries have set up (and sometimes have had in place for many years) surveys providing the necessary statistical information for preventing occupational risks.

However, considerable changes have come about in the working environment during the past twenty years or so in all industrialised countries, and this environment is undergoing the effects of pro-

---

14. Société française de santé publique (French Public Health Society), *"La pollution atmosphérique d'origine automobile et la santé publique: bilan de 15 ans de recherche internationale"* (Public health and atmospheric pollution due to cars: evaluation of 15 years of international research), Société française de santé publique, Collection Santé et Société 1996, 4, 251 p.

found alterations in each country's economy. These economic upheavals lead firms to modify their structure and organisation. They bring in novel modes of production, such as "just-in-time" manufacturing whereby finished or semi-finished products are produced just in time to be sold, transformed or assembled, "taut flow" or elimination of stocks, or "multipurpose" posts where employees are rotated between several work posts or change posts according to company requirements. Companies are incorporating new technologies and generalising work flexibility, by remunerating on an individual basis (payment according to yield, etc.), developing atypical work schedules, relying on part-time employees, subcontracting and temping.

All these transformations have important consequences on the work of employees and give rise to frequently powerful pressures: organisational pressures linked to the company and pressures which directly concern the employee, the work load, the work content, the latitude in decision-making, time constraints, social relationships in the workplace, and professional prospects. Atypical work schedules lead to fractionated, irregular work hours and disruptions in the social rhythms of employees. The need to master new technologies implies adaptation and training to cope with the increasing complexity of tasks. The development of "special forms of employment", which cover an array of diverse situations (fixed term contracts, temporary work, part-time work, assisted posts, etc.) generates vulnerability and job insecurity. In the last few years, many studies carried out in various scientific disciplines (ergonomics, psychopathology, epidemiology) have demonstrated the effects on health of pressures related to the organisation of work, particularly in the area of cardiovascular disease, mental health, and musculoskeletal conditions.

A statistical understanding of working conditions and exposure to physical, chemical and biological pollutants is a determinant factor in studying risks to health of occupational origin. The 1994 Sumer survey recently filled in most of the statistical shortcomings in this respect.

THE SUMER SURVEY*

Sumer 94* is a survey that was carried out in 1994 at the initiative of the Ministry of Employment and Solidarity by 1,200 volunteer doctors practising occupational medicine among 48,000 employees randomly chosen from those seen during the mandatory annual medical check-up. This sample of employees was comparable with the French employee population in terms of the distribution of socioprofessional categories in the employer's sector of activity and the size of the company.

The company doctor had to note the characteristics of the employee and his/her employer and, using a closed questionnaire consisting of 200 items, the organisational and physical stresses, and chemical and biological pollution present in the work place. Finally, the company doctor had to estimate the risk of disease due to the working conditions or working environment.

* Héran-Le Roy O., Sandret N., Expositions professionnelles (Occupational exposure): Sumer 94, l'état des lieux (Status report), *Santé et Travail*, 1997; 20: 13-17.

Two important public health problems related to the working environment are tackled below: one deals with periarticular disorders, and the other the effects of asbestos (for which INSERM recently prepared a scientific update[15]).

Periarticular disorders

Extent of the problem

In every country for which data are available, periarticular disorders are showing a marked increase. The list of conditions included in table 57 of occupational diseases (general scheme) entitled "periarticular conditions induced by certain work movements and postures" corresponds almost exactly to what is usually classified under the heading "periarticular disorders": tendinitis of the shoulder, of the elbow (epicondylitis, "golf elbow"), tendinitis and tendosynovitis of the wrist, tendinitis of the knee and ankle; nerve syndromes of the knee and upper limbs, including carpal tunnel syndrome; hygromas including hygroma of the knee, frequently found among those who install fitted carpets or tiling. However, traditional occupations are making a decreasingly smaller contribution to the latter condition.

The most recent data concerning occupational diseases recognised in table 57 are as follows: 3,963 (53% of occupational diseases) in 1994, 4,704 (55% of occupational diseases) in 1995, 5,856 (63% of occupational diseases) in 1996. There has been a more than 6-fold increase in frequency within the space of 10 years. The altered presentation of table 57 in 1991 had a few effects in increasing the frequency, but fails to account for it altogether since the augmentation was not restricted to the years just following 1991.

These observations and similar observations in other countries make it necessary to look primarily at changing working conditions for an explanation of these disorders, only a small fraction of which are treated as occupational diseases.

In fact, for carpal tunnel syndrome (CTS) alone, it is estimated that 130,000 surgical operations are carried out for CTS in France every year, whereas approximately 2,000 cases are recognised in table 57. Yet one study recently conducted in Montreal estimated that CTS was attributable to work in the case of 76% of men and

---

15. *"Effets sur la santé des principaux types d'exposition à l'amiante"* (Effects of main types of exposure to asbestos on health), Paris, Ed. INSERM Expertises Collectives, 1997.

55% of women among manual workers who underwent surgery for CTS.

The Estev[16] survey of more than 20,000 employees indicated that pain affecting an upper limb and causing suffering for more than 6 months concerned 14% of men aged 37, 39% of women aged 52, and intermediate percentages for other age and sex groups. For a working employee, arm pain is a predictive factor for stopping work or becoming unemployed in the next five years.

Occupational pressures and periarticular disorders

A report by "l'Agence nationale pour l'amélioration des conditions de travail" (ANACT) (National Agency for the Improvement of Working Conditions) describes an "epidemic" of periarticular disorders which occurred within several months in a firm working for a car manufacturer; they were found to be related to a rapid increase in taut flow production and the use of unsuitable means. This example is not trivial: it clearly indicates the mechanisms most often put forward to account for the increasing number of such conditions in different countries: companies have to raise production, working faster and better. Increased productivity is made possible by greater automation but does not entirely eliminate manual tasks. The latter, *e.g.* the assembly of electrical household appliances, or the cutting and packaging of meat products, oblige the employees concerned to respect deadlines in addition to the postural requirements and specificity of the movements carried out, leading to demands on muscles and tendons that overstep physiological limits.

Repetitive movements and periarticular disorders

A survey was carried out jointly in 1993-1994 by ANACT, INSERM, the "Institut national de recherche et de sécurité pour la prévention des accidents du travail et des maladies professionnelles" (INRS) (National Research and Safety Institute for the Prevention of Occupational Injuries and Diseases), the "Direction de l'animation, de la recherche, des études et des statistiques" (DARES) (Department of Mobilisation, Research and Statistics), the "Inspection médicale du travail" (Factory Medical Inspectorate), and the "Caisse centrale de la Mutualité sociale agricole" (CCMSA) (Central Branch of the Agricultural Employees' Health Insurance Agency), in 6 regions with the co-operation of 39 doctors practising occupational medicine[17]. The sample included a reference group of 337 persons, with little or no exposure to repetitive movements, and 1,420 persons exposed to repetitive

---

16. Derriennic F., Touranchet A., Volkoff S. (ed), *"Âge, travail, santé"* (Age, work, health), Questions en santé publique, Paris, Ed. INSERM, 1996.
17. *"Affections péri-articulaires des membres inférieurs et organisation du travail"* (Periarticular disorders of the lower limbs and organisation of work), Results from the national epidemiological survey, DMT INRS, 1966; 65: 13-31.

movements in various sectors: assembly-mounting (small electrical household appliances, car accessories), food industry (mainly the transformation of meat products), the garment and shoe industries, packaging, and supermarket and hypermarket cashiers. Table 9 shows the frequency of the conditions most often noted by doctors practising occupational medicine among the 1,420 persons making repetitive movements, and 337 not making such movements. "Existence of the condition" should here be taken to mean: condition established or mentioned by the doctor, at the time of the examination, whether or not involvement was bilateral; the vast majority of these conditions was not declared as an occupational disease.

Table 9 **Periarticular disorders of the upper limb**
(percentage frequency as a function of exposure to repetitive movements)

	Frequency (%)		Attributable risk[b]
	Exposed, repetitive movements	Reference group (little or no exposure)	
Single painful shoulder	28.9[a]	16.0	45
Carpal tunnel syndrome	19.3[a]	6.6	65
Epicondylitis	12.3[a]	7.9	36
Brachial plexus neuralgia	7.2	4.4	38
Golf elbow	4.0	3.5	12
Tendinitis of extensors	4.2	1.9	54
Radial styloid dysphagia	3.9	2.2	43
Tenosynovitis of flexors	3.6	2.5	30
Synovial cysts	3.0	2.5	15

a. significant difference $p < 0.05$.
b. percentage of conditions which would disappear if exposure ceased.

Some disorders, such as carpal tunnel syndrome, were both frequently present among the population and strongly linked to exposure: among employees making repetitive movements, almost two thirds (65%) of the cases of CTS would disappear if their working conditions were made similar to those of the reference group, even if the frequency in the latter group was higher than that noted in a population strictly without any occupational exposure.

Carpal tunnel syndrome (CTS) and organisation of work

As the diagram in the following page shows, many factors are involved in the aetiology of CTS.

In this case, the personal factors are sex, obesity, and the existence of certain health problems; psychological factors are also important: anxiety, in particular, might play a role by increasing the demands made on muscles. The main biomechanical determinants are the repetitive movements of hyperextension and hyperflexion of the wrist which increase the pressure in the carpal tunnel and compress the nerve.

Initially, psychosocial factors step in, including a lack of work flexibility (dependence on a machine, impossibility of adjusting the rate and amount of work, or deciding when to take breaks). In turn, these determinants depend on factors operating within the company: particular modes of organising work and production – designed to make the company more adaptable towards its clients – may greatly penalise employees, *e.g.* by reducing manufacturing deadlines and paring stocks to a bare minimum.

In conclusion, periarticular disorders have recently shown a tendency to increase. Their determinants are known to be linked to increasing company competitiveness, indicating that such conditions will not become less prevalent, and that a multidisciplinary approach should be cultivated in reflecting on the means to be employed in reconciling company productivity with employee health.

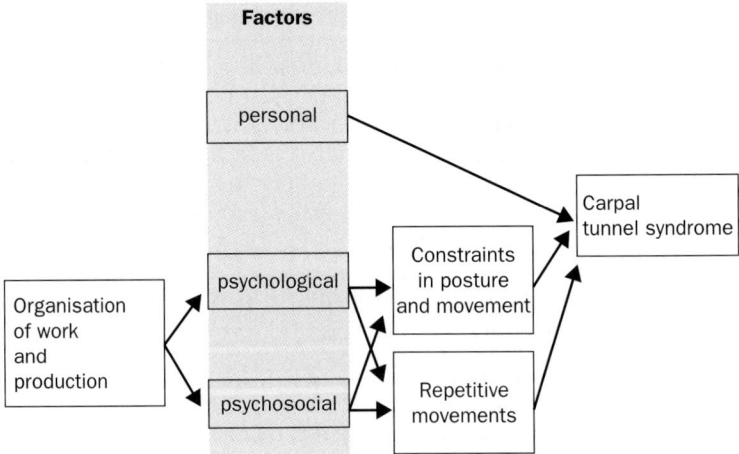

Asbestos The carcinogen present in working environments which causes by far the greatest number of cancer cases is asbestos. And yet, up until recently, very few studies had been carried out in France concerning the frequency and conditions of exposure to this pollutant and its effects on health. A collective expert appraisal by INSERM was published in July 1996, reviewing and updating knowledge on the subject, and the data below are taken from this report.

Asbestos fibres are minerals with very unusual physical and chemical properties: they do not burn, they are remarkably resistant to various aggressive chemicals, and they exhibit strong mechanical resistance. These properties have encouraged the increasing use of many forms of asbestos fibres for the manufacture of numerous, widely employed industrial products or for the construction of buildings. There are basically two varieties of asbestos: chrysotile and amphiboles.

Principal uses

The most frequently used asbestos-based material is asbestos cement, which accounts for the main part of world tonnage (65-70% of total tonnage). Apart from numerous products used in the construction industry, asbestos has been used in the form of flocking intended to increase the fire resistance of structures or to improve sound insulation. Aside from the construction industry, a broad range of sectors have turned to asbestos for less extensive but equally varied uses: cartons and paper, textiles, then friction linings and joints, and finally highly miscellaneous products (toys, items for smokers, filters for liquids, pavement products, air filters, finished textiles, and certain articles for domestic use, *e.g.* ironing boards and covers, toasters, insulating boards for do-it-yourself work and mobile heating equipment).

Main situations involving exposure to asbestos

The vast majority of cases in which the effects of asbestos on health have been established have involved occupational exposure. The people concerned produced asbestos in a working environment (extraction and transformation), used it directly for various operations of transformation (textile, Fibrociment, etc.) or heat or sound insulation, or handled asbestos-containing materials. Such materials are very often handled, particularly in the construction industry, and it has been estimated that 20% of 60-year-old men in industrialised countries have been exposed to asbestos at least once during the course of their professional career.

Environmental exposure may be classified into three categories, depending on the source of pollution:
– pollution emitted by a "natural" source (geological site) in certain regions where the soil contains asbestos fibres which are inhaled as people breathe during the course of various activities;
– pollution emitted by a specific "industrial" source (asbestos mine, plant for asbestos transformation) which discharges asbestos fibres into the surroundings where they may be inhaled by persons living or working in the environment;
– pollution emitted by asbestos fitted in buildings and various installations, and whose fibres may be released into the atmosphere, either due to degradation or manipulation of the installations.
The concentration of fibres in the atmosphere varies greatly : it may be high in a working environment (from about one fibre per millilitre of air (f/ml) to about one fibre per litre of air (f/l)), and even markedly less than one f/l in urban settings or undegraded flocked premises.

CHANGES IN THE REGULATIONS CONCERNING ASBESTOS IN FRANCE AND ABROAD

The carcinogenicity of asbestos was scientifically proven in the 1950s but it was not until 1977 that France, like most European countries, adopted regulations to protect workers, and then the general population. At that time, the aim was to "control" the use of asbestos, in spite of lively debate as to whether any use could realistically be guaranteed free from risk.

A distinction must be made between three different types of asbestos utilisation, each governed by specific regulations.

Limits for worker exposure to asbestos dust were first established in 1977 and have consistently been tightened since then as a result of successive European directives. In 1996, France went even further by adopting stricter limits than those decided by the European directive of 25 January 1991, which is still in effect (see table).

Asbestos flocking was prohibited in France in 1977 for housing, and then in 1978 for all buildings if the asbestos concentration in the products used was greater than 1%. The discharge of asbestos by flocking, and activities involving insulating or soundproofing materials with a density of less than 1 g/cm^3 were banned in 1992.

In the case of asbestos-containing products, France was initially content to apply the European directives before going further and prohibiting them entirely. The ban was carried out in three stages, bearing in mind the carcinogenicity of the different varieties of asbestos:
– in 1988, one variety of asbestos, crocidolite, was prohibited (with three exceptions);
– in 1994, the marketing, utilisation and importation of all amphiboles were prohibited. Only chrysotile remained authorised, apart from certain products;
– in 1996, decree No. 96-1133 of 24 December prohibited the manufacture, importation, marketing, exportation and sale of all varieties of asbestos, although a few special dispensations were allowed.

	Exposure limits		Ban on flocking	Ban on products
	Chrysotile	Others		
European Union	0.6 f/ml	0.3 f/ml		controlled use
France	0.1 f/ml	0.1 f/ml	1977/1978	prohibited on 24 December 1996
Belgium	0.5 f/ml	0.15 f/ml	1980	controlled use
United Kingdom	0.6 f/ml	0.2 f/ml	1985	controlled use
Germany	0.15 f/ml	0.15 f/ml	1979	prohibited in 1979 over 10 years
Spain	0.6 f/ml	0.3 f/ml		controlled use
Switzerland	0.25 f/ml	0.25 f/ml	1975	prohibited on 1 September 1986

Protection regulations

Since the first statutory measures were introduced in the United Kingdom in 1931, there has been a gradual reduction in the permissible maximum limits for occupational exposure promulgated in many countries. At a later date, the use of certain forms of asbestos was prohibited in some countries, and any form of asbestos in others. At the same time, statutory measures were adopted for so-called "passive" exposure encountered in buildings. From the 1960s onwards, the flocking of buildings was extensively carried out, but was banned in France in 1978. The regulations adopted in 1996 stipulate that exposure to 5 f/l or less is permissible in buildings, that corrective work must be instigated when the level of exposure is greater than or equal to 25 f/l, and that intermediate levels require intensified surveillance.

Risks to health associated with asbestos exposure

The beginning of the century saw a considerable increase in the production and industrial use of asbestos. In subsequent decades, there was a major "epidemic" of pulmonary fibrosis, lung cancer and mesotheliomas. Other locations of asbestos-related cancer have also been mentioned in the literature.

The risk of pulmonary fibrosis, known as "asbestosis", was the first to have been established (in 1906) and various forms of benign pleural involvement have also been associated with exposure to asbestos, the most frequent being pleural plaques.

The initial report suggesting the existence of a link between occupational exposure to asbestos and the risk of lung cancer was published in 1935. In 1955, after repeated confirmation and using a method for the first time regarded as rigorous, R. Doll demonstrated that occupational exposure to asbestos was responsible for an increased risk of lung cancer among a population of textile asbestos workers in the United Kingdom. In 1977, the "Centre international de recherche sur le cancer" (CIRC) (International Cancer Research Centre) classified asbestos in the category of "agents carcinogenic in man", and it has been clearly established that the causal relationship between exposure to asbestos and lung cancer also holds true among non smokers. The mean latent period between exposure and the onset of the disease is several decades. It is estimated that 5 to 7% of cases of lung cancer among men in industrialised countries can be attributed to occupational exposure to asbestos.

The first pointers to the existence of a risk of mesothelioma associated with exposure to asbestos were observed in 1960 among miners of crocidolite in South Africa. It also very quickly became apparent that there was a risk of mesothelioma in the textile asbestos sector, and a particularly high risk among manual workers in dockyards and among those installing heat insulation. In 1977, the CIRC regarded asbestos as carcinogenic in man, also because of the increased risk of mesothelioma. Mesotheliomas are primarily located in the pleura, pleural mesothelioma being on the whole five times more frequent than peritoneal mesothelioma, other locations very rarely being affected. The average latent period between exposure and the onset of the disease is between 30 and 40 years. Except for exposure to asbestos, there is currently no known risk factor associated with mesothelioma. All the evidence seems to agree in imputing almost all cases of mesothelioma in industrialised countries to occupational exposure to asbestos. As with the example of lung cancer, the evidence indicates that every type of asbestos fibre, including chrysotile, is capable of inducing mesotheliomas.

A considerable change in the occupations affected has occurred over the last few decades, and most cases of mesothelioma are nowadays encountered in industrialised countries in very varied trades. In the 1960s, it should be recalled that the main occupations affected were those which involved asbestos manufacture and utilisation: workers in the insulation sector, asbestos production and transformation, those carrying out heating installation, and dockyard workers. In contrast, the most affected trades in the 1980s and 1990s were sheet-iron workers and boiler makers (category including dockyard workers), and industrial carriage-builders; these were followed by plumbers, carpenters and electricians. Building trades alone currently account for one quarter of all deaths due to mesothelioma, and it is felt that this is probably an underestimate. As an example, among the trades at high risk of mesothelioma may be mentioned those as diverse as welders, dockers, laboratory technicians, painters and decorators, jewellers, adjusters, car mechanics, railroad workers, etc. The levels of exposure are probably lower than in the past, but these trades employ large numbers of workers and this explains why a great many cases of mesothelioma have been observed. In addition, since these trades are not usually considered to be "at risk", they are subject to less surveillance and fewer measures aimed at adequate protection.

As far as passive exposure inside buildings is concerned, no epidemiological data currently exist that would answer the question of whether it poses a potential risk.

There are various methodological reasons that account for the absence of such data, particularly the fact that in any case the risk could only be small (this type of exposure is characterized by usually very low average concentrations of fibres), and that so far the follow-up period in studying the risk of mesothelioma has been too short: exposure related to physical presence in asbestos-containing buildings is actually relatively recent since the widespread use of asbestos for heat and sound insulation in buildings began in the 1960s, while the mean latent period for pleural mesothelioma is estimated to be 30 to 40 years.

Data concerning variations in the incidence of mesothelioma

An analysis of changes in the incidence of mesothelioma among men in industrialised countries shows that a real pandemic started in the 1950s and has been progressing at the rate of about 5 to 10% per year since then. The pandemic and its dynamics are closely linked to the introduction and greatly increasing use of asbestos in industrialised countries which began in most at the end of the first World War. In all countries, a time-lag of 30 to 40 years has been noted between the initial use of asbestos for industrial purposes and the start of the progressive epidemic of mesotheliomas. Depending on the country concerned, a few differences have been observed in the dynamics of the epidemic, related to the initial period of asbestos introduction and the nature of the fibres employed. Australia and South Africa used mainly crocidolite − with its strongly associated risk of mesothelioma − and recently attained the highest incidence of mesothelioma in industrialised countries, ranging from 40 to almost 70 times the rate expected in the absence of any exposure to asbestos.

On the whole, the situation in France is comparable to that in other industrialised countries, but with certain specific features. In the period 1968-1992, the augmentation in the incidence of mesothelioma was constant and stable among both men and women, but the rate of increase was greater among men: the annual mean increase was 3.8% for the entire population (4.3% among men and 2.8% among women).

Over a shorter period (1979-1990), data derived from cancer registers show a multiplication factor for men, relative to the period 1979-1981, of 1.7 in 1982-1984 and of 2.2 in 1988-1990.

Based on the estimated incidence of mesothelioma and its progression, and the fraction of lung cancers attributable to occupational exposure to asbestos (this datum is unavailable in France, but was estimated at 5.7% for the current period in the United Kingdom and has been used here), it has been estimated that the number of deaths in 1996 attributable in France to asbestos exposure was about 1950 (750 due to mesothelioma and 1,200 due to lung cancer); the vast majority, if not all, of these deaths were undeniably the result of occupational or para-occupational exposure to asbestos. It should be stressed that this estimate expresses the minimum value for the actual number of deaths imputable to asbestos, since the fraction of mesotheliomas (and lung cancers) which escape any medical diagnosis cannot be evaluated.

Epidemiological data compiled from fifteen or so studies can be used to establish a suitable model to describe the risk of mortality due to lung cancer attributable to asbestos in populations subjected to continuous occupational exposure to high levels of asbestos fibres (from 1 f/ml to more than 200 f/ml) as a function of the level of exposure. In measuring the excess mortality due to mesothelioma, the only available data come from three studies on populations exposed to high levels in the course of their work. There are no methods which allow direct, positive measurement of the risks of lung cancer and mesothelioma in human populations exposed to low levels: hence, such risks at low levels can only be estimated by extrapolating from models worked out for high levels of occupational exposure. The extrapolated results are not scientifically valid but are useful in contemplating how to control risks: in our present state of knowledge, this uncertain method of estimating is the most plausible for the moment. Table 10 shows the risks that have been estimated in this way: they correspond to current reference levels as per French regulations. They indicate the additional number of cases of lung cancer and mesothelioma attributable to continuous exposure to asbestos from the time of initial exposure up until the age of 80 as a function of the age at which exposure began and finished, and as a function of the level of exposure.

Table 10 **Estimated number of additional deaths due to lung cancer and mesothelioma up until the age of 80 attributable to "continuous" exposure to asbestos as a function of the level of exposure (f/ml) and sex**

Level (f/ml)	Exposure from 20 to 65 years		Exposure from 5 to 65 years	
	Men	Women	Men	Women
1	+3.1 / 100	+1.6 / 100	+6.0 / 100	+4.1 / 100
0.1	+3.1 / 1,000	+1.6 / 1,000	+6.0 / 1,000	+4.1 / 1,000
0.025	+0.8 / 1,000	+0.4 / 1,000	+1.5 / 1,000	+1.0 / 1,000
0.01	+3.1 / 10,000	+1.6 / 10,000	+6.0 / 10,000	+4.1 / 10,000
0.001	+3.1 / 100,000	+1.6 / 100,000	+6.0 / 100,000	+4.1 / 100,000

These deaths are in addition to the expected deaths due to lung cancer and mesothelioma up until the age of 80 per thousand persons (51 men and 7 women).
Reading: Continuous exposure to 0.1 f/ml of asbestos between the ages of 20 to 65 years gives rise to 3.1 additional cases of lung cancer or mesothelioma before the age of 80 per thousand men exposed, *i.e.* mean = 54.1 cases.
a. 40 h/week x 48 weeks/year = 1 920 per year.
Source: Inserm.

Table 10 shows that statutory stipulation of the limit values (0.1 f/ml for occupational exposure and 0.025 f/ml for intramural exposure) ensures that a large fraction of potentially exposed persons are actually exposed to levels far below the reference values and for limited time periods. However, some people are certainly exposed to higher concentrations and for longer periods. It should be emphasised that, because of a lack of suitable data, major uncertainties exist. It is therefore impossible at the present time to extrapolate these estimates for 10,000 exposed individuals to find the number of cases attributable to asbestos exposure on a national scale.

Compensation for occupational diseases

Payments made within the scope of French legislation for work-related ill health concern actual "occupational injuries", "journey injuries", and "occupational diseases". This social coverage is provided for all employees and comparable categories, its aim being to reimburse health care costs caused by the injury or disease and also a fraction (usually very limited) of lost income. Recent changes in the frequency of occupational injuries liable for compensation have been described above. The problems posed by according recognition to "occupational diseases" are mentioned below.

In the French system, any condition induced by a physical, chemical or microbial toxic agent is only recognised as "occupational" if it is explicitly listed in a table of "occupational diseases" in existence at the time of its declaration. This is a necessary – but insufficient – condition since other criteria must also be satisfied at the same time. If the condition does not arise when the worker is still exposed to the risk, it must be medically observed within a time interval known as the "délai de prise en charge" (reimbursement deadline). The victim must also provide "evidence" of his "usual" exposure to the risk. In some cases, the work performed by the victim must be explicitly mentioned in a "closed" list of work said to be solely responsible for inducing the occupational disease considered. For certain tables, special conditions are added to these general provisions, e.g. a minimum duration of exposure to the toxic agent inducing the condition. The victim (or the victim's legal representative) must make the administrative declaration of his condition to the social security organisation concerned.

Variation in the number of recognised occupational diseases

The present compensation system was created by the law of 25 October 1919, and was particularly expanded from 1946 onwards (26 tables in 1946 and 106 today). For several years, about 4,000 cases of recognised occupational diseases per year were officially registered. The statistical data presented relate to employees in the general social security system which covers about 80% of employees.

The first appreciable change in the number of recognised conditions was noted in 1983-1984. Following a significant alteration in the criteria for considering occupational hearing loss, there was practically a 5-fold increase in the number of cases of recognised hearing loss; the effect subsequently wore off. The second important modification in the number of recognised conditions began in 1991-1992 and was due to better reimbursement for periarticular disorders induced primarily by repetitive movements. Since then, the number of recognised conditions has continued to increase. The mean annual number of conditions recognised in 1995 was practically double that recognised between 1955 and 1990.

The recognition of asbestos-induced injuries has also significantly increased since the beginning of the 1990s because of the relatively long latent period for so-called benign involvement and even longer for cancerous conditions. However, the extent of occupational injuries is very poorly reflected by the number of recognised diseases, as was especially shown by the recent collective expert appraisal by INSERM.

Figure 12 shows the comparative changes in the total number of recognised occupational diseases and all of those recognised in the 5 tables which have progressively played a major role in the system of recognition (69% of recognised diseases in 1993-1995).

Figure 12 **Comparative variations in recognised occupational diseases and those shown in tables 8, 25, 42, 45 and 47**

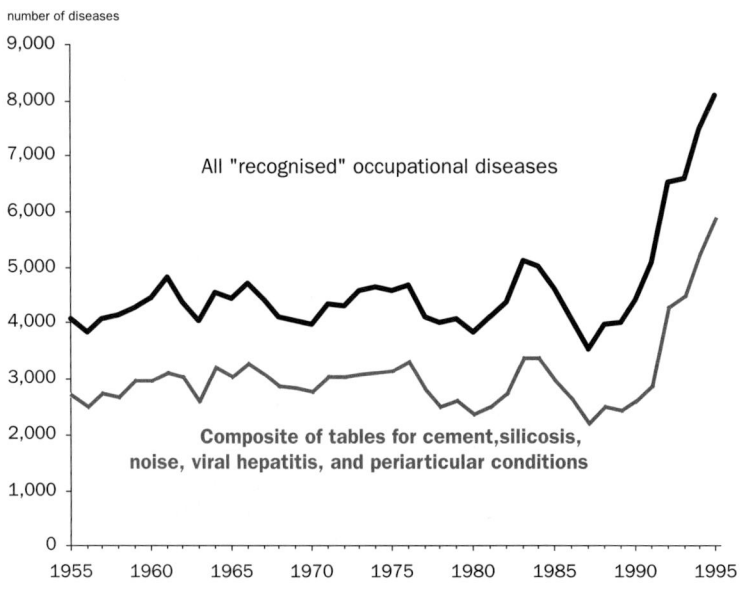

Source: Cnamts.

Geographic disparities in recognition

The Deniel report[18] underlined the pronounced regional differences which existed in the number of recognised occupational diseases. The anticipated number of occupational diseases was calculated so as to compare it with the corresponding number observed in 1995, assuming that each industrial sector has the same mean rate of recognition at the regional and national levels. Table 11 shows the appreciable differences in several regions between the number of predicted recognised diseases and those actually observed.

Table 11 **Comparison of the number of occupational diseases "acknowledged" by the Regional Branches of the National Health Insurance Agency in 1995 and the "expected" number of diseases**

	Observed	Expected	Difference
Bordeaux	202	354	– 75%
Clermont-Ferrand	133	182	– 37%
Dijon	458	420	8%
Lille	602	836	– 39%
Limoges	292	304	– 4%
Lyon	818	915	– 12%
Marseille	413	520	– 26%
Montpellier	134	220	– 64%
Nancy	481	387	20%
Nantes	1,059	494	53%
Orléans	437	377	14%
Paris	1,121	1,788	– 59%
Rennes	861	358	58%
Rouen	612	467	24%
Strasbourg	560	450	20%
Toulouse	197	307	– 56%
Total	8,380	8,380	0%

Various explanations might be suggested to account for the very marked geographical divergences. However, it would be necessary to know the number of persons who submit a request for recognition and the number of dossiers accepted as a function of each table of occupational diseases and each CRAM. Surprisingly, these data are not available and the statistics presently published do not give a clear picture of the actual situation. Nor do they allow the administration and management and labour to assess the relevance of the current system of compensation.

International comparisons reveal that the French situation is worrying as far as the recognition of occupational diseases is concerned. French employees are at a disadvantage compared with

---

18. Report to the Government by the Deniel Commission within the framework of the law on financing of "sécurité sociale" in 1997.

Part two Changes in health status

employees in other European countries and this is illustrated by the example of asbestos-induced diseases (table 12).

Table 12 **Comparison of the occupational disease rates acknowledged as asbestos-induced in Germany, Belgium and France**
(cumulative rate per million inhabitants for the period 1984-1993)

	Germany	Belgium	France
Asbestosis	65.6	170.9	30.9
Lung cancer	21.1	6.0	2.0
Mesothelioma	39.1	28.1	7.6
Death	50.9	30.3	3.8

Even if the various countries compared have dissimilar recognition systems, this cannot account for such wide differences, nor can they be explained by saying that the risks are much lower in France, given that French mortality rates due to pleural carcinoma are similar in magnitude to those in other European countries.

The complementary system

In 1993-1994, a complementary system was set up whereby dossiers for occupational diseases which had been rejected at the first reading (because one or more criteria were not met), even though the declared condition was listed in one of the tables, were included in a "second chance" system: this supplied an undeniable "breath of oxygen". However, very little compensation is paid by the complementary system for diseases not yet listed in any of the tables – the victim either has to be incapable of any type of work or dead. In the first 18 months (1994-1995), 609 cases were recognised out of the 1,086 dossiers submitted for a "second chance", *i.e.* a recognition rate of 56%. 72% of the recognised cases were covered by just three tables: table 57 relating to "periarticular disorders" (44%), table 42 concerning "occupational hearing loss" (20%), and table 66 concerning "allergic respiratory conditions" (8%). However, of 99 dossiers involving an occupational condition unlisted in any of the tables, only 25 (25%) were recognised.

The example of mortality due to work-related cancer

Accessible mortality data only deal with the 14.5 million employees in the 1995 general system out of a national working population at that time of 25.3 million, *i.e.* 6 out of 10 workers.

In the last year for which figures are available, 1995, 253 deaths due to occupational diseases listed in the set of 102 existing tables were recognised, whereas compensation was awarded for 1,430 deaths due to occupational injuries and work-related journeys. Currently accepted estimates put the figure for deaths due to work-related cancer at 5% of all deaths due to cancer: for 1994 (144,746 deaths due to cancer in France), the lowest estimate therefore puts the number of work-related cancer deaths at about 5,800; for asbestos-induced deaths alone in 1996, the INSERM collective expert appraisal already mentioned gave an estimate of a minimum of 1950. Although there has been an increase in the number of recognised cancers in recent years, the vast majority are still ignored: assuming that the 253 deaths recognised as being due to occupational diseases in 1995 were cancer-related, the mortality due to work-related cancer would, for workers covered by the general system (14.5 million employees), therefore be underestimated by a factor of at least 13 (figure 13).

Figure 13 **Variation in the total number of cases of work-related cancer recognised annually in France**

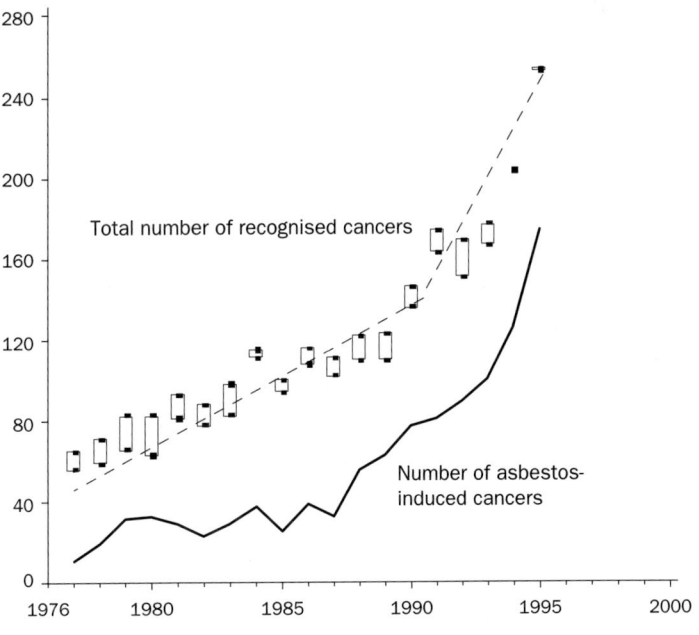

Source: Cnamts.

CHAPTER FIVE

Overview

General indicators

During the period 1991-1996, the **general indicators** of mortality and life expectancy continued to progress since, for an identical age structure, the population's mortality rate dropped by 6% and its life expectancy at birth increased by 11 months. However, the mean annual variation was lower than during the period 1981-1991, since the reduction in mortality among those over 65 years of age had marked time during the more recent period.

In contrast, considerable gains in **avoidable premature mortality** were noted for both sexes, whether for reasons particularly linked to lifestyle (– 21%) or the medical care and screening system (– 11%). This observation is all the more important, given that France is characterised by very high avoidable excess premature mortality relative to other European countries. However, as the comparison between France and England-and-Wales in the present report shows, the favourable progress made in France during the period 1991-1996 is not sufficient to significantly close the gap. The same is true for the **indicators of excess mortality**: these are particularly high in France, such as excess male mortality or inter-regional differences in excess mortality and have remained stable on the whole.

The advantage of analysing global indicators which encompass both mortality and morbidity data was clearly demonstrated in the 1994 HCSP report, thanks to the calculation of life expectancy with and without unimpaired health. The prolongation of **life expectancy with unimpaired health** during the period 1981-1991 (slightly longer than that of total life expectancy) indicated not only quantitative but also qualitative progress in survival.

No study could be made of recent changes in this indicator since there are no available comparable data for the prevalence of disability in France over the period 1991-1996. In the future, it will probably be necessary to repeat surveys – such as the INSEE decennial health survey – more frequently so as to improve global indicator monitoring.

Part two — Changes in health status

Specific indicators

An analysis of changes in the **specific indicators** of problems and priority health determinants defined in the 1994 HCSP report could have been carried out independently of the **development targets** which had been set for some of them. However, it seemed to be of interest to compare them with the changes actually observed since their publication. The comparison is purely indicative since the targets were expressed in many ways (quantified or otherwise), and had been worked out in different manners (by simple "extrapolation" in some cases, and by "characterised voluntarism" in others). Nevertheless, it is the first time that such an experiment has been conducted in the area of health in France.

In the following overview, indicators have been grouped into three categories depending on the direction of the changes undergone during the last period. In most cases, the changes indicate that public health actions must be implemented or continued, though obviously a detailed analysis of the latter is beyond the scope of the present report.

The problems of **vulnerability and social integration** and the questions of **access to care and prevention** among disadvantaged populations show a strong association with the economic climate (job insecurity, etc.) and the political context (reform of social protection, etc.), both of which have undergone some shifts in the past five years. The High Committee on Public Health gave detailed consideration to these subjects and issued appropriate recommendations in a report made public in 1998[1].

Deteriorating health

- Based on comparisons with other countries and the rising consumption of tobacco over the last ten years or so, an increase in the incidence and mortality due to **lung cancer** and **cancers and of the upper airways and digestive tract** among women had been widely anticipated and predicted; it became a patent epidemiological fact in the period 1991-1996. Absolute rates are still low compared with those observed in men, though this is obviously not an argument for putting off the necessary measures to prevent smoking. Such actions, probably both general and specific, should limit extension of the predicted epidemic of these types of cancer among women over the next few years if no attempt is made to change course.
- The sustained increase in incidence and mortality due to **melanoma** in both sexes over the period 1991-1996 clearly indicates that prevention has been a failure and this must be corrected.

---

1. *"La progression de la précarité en France et ses effets sur la santé"* (Increasing vulnerability in France and its effects on health), HCSP report by a working party presided over by J.-D. Rainhorn, February 1998, Rennes: Ed. ENSP, 1998, 368 p.

Overview

- Although changes in all indicators concerning **at-risk behaviour among the young and adolescents** are far from unsatisfactory, some of the changes noted in behaviour are causing much disquiet, especially those involving the consumption of psychoactive substances. It can never be sufficiently stressed that the idea of prevention makes the most sense and is doubtless most effective among the young and adolescents. The importance of education in the family and then school in determining health in young adults has been specifically analysed in the report *"Santé des enfants, santé des jeunes"* (Health in children and young people) published by the HCSP in 1997[2].

A renewal of the topics and form of messages of prevention aimed at the young appears to be required over the short term, in addition to the mandatory medium- and long-term initiatives which have either been taken or will be taken in this connection.

Unchanging health

- During the period 1991-1996, the mortality rate due to **suicide** (and probably the frequency of attempted suicide) saw only a small decline, and even increased among men aged 15 to 44.

The National health conference, and several regional conferences and regional health programmes identified suicide as a priority health problem. Considerable effort will probably be needed to combat this scourge effectively.

- Between 1990 and 1995, there was practically no change in the mortality rate due to **breast cancer** whereas there was a 16% rise in the incidence of the disease. These results indicate that its management has improved, thanks to earlier diagnosis and more effective treatment, and they demonstrate the advantage of more rapid, rational screening and also of finding means of effective primary prevention. The situation is not dissimilar from that of **colorectal cancer** where the mortality rate (especially among the under 65s) has fallen slightly but the incidence has increased by 13%. Yet again, primary prevention must be given priority in the future.
- The mortality and incidence of **lung cancer** appears to have reached a plateau among men. The fight against smoking must be kept up and should lead to a lower incidence of lung cancer in the future.
- **Perinatal mortality** saw a regular decline up until 1992 and has remained stable since then. The prematurity rate appears to have slightly increased during the period 1988-1995 and the proportion of birth weights under 2,500 g has remained constant. It should be remembered that a national perinatal action programme

---

2. High Committee on Public Health. *"Santé des enfants, santé des jeunes"* (Health among children and young people), Paris, HCSP, 1997, 158 p. Report by a working party presided over irsch.

has been under way since 1994. In addition, **maternal mortality** has not shown any decrease recently and special measures will be required, involving an automatic medical audit.

- Declarations of **back pain** by the population have remained relatively stable over the last few years although it is more frequently the reason why patients consult their doctor. Combined action should doubtless be taken to initiate experimental preventive procedures and to develop references to help guide the diagnosis and medical management.

Improving health

It goes without saying that there can be no slackening of effort once positive changes in an indicator have been obtained without this having a deleterious effect. A good illustration is provided by the changes in two essential determinants of health, *i.e.* tobacco and alcohol consumption. While it is true that average consumptions among the entire population dropped during the period 1991-1996, a) they remain at a high level and the decline has to continue, b) consumption has increased among some sections of the population, c) the reduction was not uniform throughout the period and there has been no change over the last few years.

All of these reasons point to the need for maintaining an active policy of prevention aimed at both the demand and supply of the product. In the case of the battle against excessive alcohol consumption, there is a particular need for a coherent, overall plan which defines responsibilities and covers the means required for treatment and rehabilitation.

- Comparative mortality rates due to **accidents of daily life** dropped by 14% between 1991 and 1996, as did the number of hospital admissions related to such accidents. Efforts aimed at prevention must be intensified and diversified, bearing in mind that accidents are age-specific.
- The number of **road accidents involving bodily injury**, and the numbers of killed and injured, have been declining since 1988, though a slowdown has been clearly apparent in the last few years. The differences in mortality relative to other European countries are as large as ever. Some progress has been noted in driving behaviour (wearing a seat belt, determination of the blood alcohol concentration in the case of accidents), but the number of speeding offences has remained constant. New provisions are set out in the draft bill on road safety which is being passed.
- The frequency of **occupational injuries** which led to time off work, and their mean severity in terms of permanent disability, have decreased since 1991 when the number of hours worked is taken into account, even though there is a tendency not to declare accidents of a less serious nature. Obviously, renewed preventive efforts must be made so that the decline continues, although

some aspects of changing working conditions (schedules, temporary work, etc.) are not very conducive *a priori* to reducing injuries.
- There was a continued drop in total **cardiovascular mortality** due to ischaemic heart disease and cerebrovascular disease for both sexes between 1991 and 1996, although at a slower rate than in the previous five years. Available data concerning infarction (1985-1993) indicate that there was a smaller decline in the incidence of infarction than in that of coronary mortality. The result shows the progress that has been made in the medical management of patients suffering from coronary insufficiency and the importance of maintaining a primary prevention policy for cardiovascular diseases in the future.
- The policy of preventing the risks of sexual and intravenous contamination by HIV led to a decrease in the number of new cases of **AIDS** from 1994 onwards; since 1996, this has been helped by advances made using triple therapies. A marked decrease in the incidence of **sexually transmitted diseases** has also been noted.
- A substantial fall in **infantile mortality** has been obtained, thanks to the prevention of sudden death in infants under one year old, so that France is approaching the levels observed in Scandinavian countries for this indicator.

Having rapidly reviewed the principal indicators analysed in the report, it would be worthwhile to make some additional comments.

Health and the environment

The importance of health and the environment was announced in the 1994 HCSP report and has manifestly become a public health concern in the last five years. The public and the media are particularly aware of pollution and the physical environment and their effects on health. It is vital that the terms of inevitable future debates on this topic remain scientific, and the High Committee on Public Health has therefore sought to introduce the subject in as instructive a manner as possible by analysing two examples which show that, although there are many scientific imponderables, a rational basis must nevertheless be used in arriving at public health decisions. The long-term effects of atmospheric pollution, and the effects of low dose-exposure to asbestos illustrate this approach. Introducing a discussion on occupational diseases provides an opportunity for issuing a reminder that the effect of environmental factors can most often be observed in the workplace, and yet the recognition of their responsibility continues to pose serious problems, particularly in France.

Poor standards for measuring health

How can one ignore the paradox created by the wish to adopt a broad, positive notion of health when the indicators employed most often concern specific diseases and generally only refer to the mortality they induce? The estimates of morbidity due to cancer or myocardial infarction given in the present report clearly constitute an advance, but it must be stressed that they are difficult to obtain and it is not simple to extend the structure of the morbidity register to other diseases. Moreover, the report has shown that there are limitations to interpreting changes in the data pertaining to morbidity as stated by the individuals themselves. The same would have been true if data concerning variations in hospital morbidity had been available for the period considered. It is likely that similar difficulties will restrict the use of data derived from the PMSI in the future. What will happen when all of the health sectors have been computerised?

From another point of view, perhaps progress could be made by measuring the effects of good or poor health in functional, psychological, etc. terms by means of repeated surveys which are as standardised as possible. It is also essential that such data should be comparable on an international scale. Immense scope for inter-institutional co-operation has been opened up concerning the development of health indicators, and it was doubtless the intention of legislators to organise such co-operation when it gave the Health Surveillance Institute responsibility for monitoring health in France.

PART THREE

A few organisational problems in the health system

INTRODUCTION

A few organisational problems in the health system

Nowadays, it is accepted that the responsibility for health policy is exerted essentially in three ways: by protecting health (ensuring safety and surveillance), promoting health (encouraging behaviour conducive to good health), and organising medical care. More generally, questions concerning the organisation of the health system so as to make it more efficient play a vital role and the way they unfold has a major influence on the balance-sheet which can be drawn up for indicators and determinants. For the third part of the report, the decision was taken to analyse three problems encountered in different sectors of the health system: the early detection of cancers affecting women, emergency treatment in hospitals, and allowances for elderly dependent persons – the need to make progress for the latter has been generally agreed for several years past but the problem has yet to be satisfactorily resolved. Without doubt, the links between these three examples should make it easier to appreciate some of the difficulties in the health system and point out the direction in which changes should be made.

CHAPTER SIX

Screening for female cancers in France

In its 1994 report, *Health in France*, the High Committee on Public Health stressed the major imbalance between expenditure on medical care and expenditure on prevention. In terms of cancer prevention, screening could, if organised under good conditions, reduce mortality, thanks to the earlier treatment of cases which have been screened and then diagnosed. This is particularly true for breast cancer and cervical cancer.

The extent to which such tests are organised among the public primarily determines the degree of effectiveness which can be expected. In fact, effectiveness depends on the level of coverage among the population, compliance with screening at defined intervals, quality control of the tests carried out, and appropriate management of those whose results are abnormal.

Slow progress has been made in generalising screening for such cancers and this is probably due to the difficulty of reconciling the performance of tests in the general interest with the individual approach that normally prevails in the French medical care system.

Screening for cancer raises many methodological, technical, and also ethical problems, related to adherence to a specific, rigorous programme – this can sometimes give rise to appreciable iatrogenic repercussions since they then affect people who are in good health. It is, in fact, of the utmost importance to ensure that the expected benefits in terms of reduced mortality or morbidity outweigh the risks or side effects linked to the screening process itself, to the additional tests carried out if screening gives a positive result, and the psychological effects of these procedures.

Cervical cancer and breast cancer are two examples of conditions that have been allocated specific means for screening over the past few years.

Screening for cervical cancer

Statistical estimates based on data from French cancer registers[1] reveal that a substantial decrease has occurred in cases of cervical cancer. They have fallen successively in number from 6,000 in 1975, to 4,200 in 1985, and 3,300 in 1995. At the same time, the number of deaths fell from 2,500 in 1985 to 1,630 in 1995, more than 80% of the women being over 50. Part of the decreased incidence and mortality appears to be attributable to the practice of performing smears for the early detection of pre-cancerous lesions or non invasive cancer. Another explanatory factor might be the extra protection against gynaecological infections backed up by anti-AIDS campaigns[1].

In Metropolitan France, the annual incidence of cervical cancer is said to be 20 per 100,000 among women aged 35 to 49, 33 per 100,000 for those aged 50 to 64, and 35 per 100,000 for those aged 65 to 69[2]. The standardised incidence of invasive cancer fell between 1978 and 1992 from 15.6 per 100,000 to 8.6 per 100,000[1].

Several reports and expert consensuses (Lille in 1990; HCSP in 1993; ANDEM in 1994; CNC in 1996) have concluded that one smear every three years is adequate for systematic screening. According to one study carried out in 1986 by the International Cancer Research Centre based on eleven different national programmes, it should theoretically reduce specific mortality by more than 90%. In countries where organised mass screening is carried out, the mortality rates due to uterine cancer have dropped by 50 to 80%.

However, in spite of the large number of smears performed annually in France (6 to 7 million), this hypothetical situation is far from having been achieved. In fact, most articles on screening for cervical cancer note that many women have never had a smear, and some hospital series of invasive cancer cases indicate that 85 to 90% of the women had never had a smear, or had had a smear more than three years earlier.

According to the Health Barometer of the CFES, for which a sample of one thousand women were questioned in December 1995, only 8.7% had never had a smear, whereas almost 75% had had a smear less than three years earlier. Among women over 60, approximately 40% had never had a smear, or no recent smear.

---

1. C. Weidmann, P. Schaffer, G. Hedelin, P. Arveux, et al., "L'incidence du cancer du col de l'utérus régresse régulièrement en France" (The incidence of cancer of the cervix is declining regularly in France), *BEH*, 1998, No. 5, pp. 17-19.
2. De Vathaire F., Koscielny F., Rezvani A, et al., In *"Statistiques de santé"* (Health statistics). "Estimation de l'incidence des cancers en France 1983-1987" (Estimated incidence of cancer in France 1983-1987), Paris, INSERM, 1996, pp. 60-61.

The women who had not had a smear taken, other than those over 60, were mainly those who did not go out to work, or who lived in a rural setting, or who were in the artisan-shopkeeper sector; women were less likely to have had a smear if a general practitioner was responsible for their gynaecological follow-up rather than a gynaecologist. Hence, information concerning the value of screening for cervical cancer should primarily be given to such women and general practitioners.

Quality of smears

A smear is the key examination carried out in screening for cervical cancer, and the quality of the sample and the way it is obtained and interpreted all affect the global results.

From this point of view, some studies have noted false negatives ranging up to 30%. The "Agence nationale d'accréditation et d'évaluation en santé" (ANAES) (National Agency for Health Accreditation and Evaluation) has just published recommendations[3] concerning the approach to be adopted for abnormal cervical smears. The recommendations deal with all stages of the smear – sampling, cytologic methods and interpretation of results, and the statistical significance in terms of sensitivity and specificity.

As far as sampling is concerned, an improvement in quality requires that sampling should include all the ectocervix and the endocervix. The sample must be spread in an even, thin layer over the slide and fixed immediately. The techniques used in the cytologic examination actually depend on the sample being of good quality.

The Papanicolaou classification has been universally abandoned and the ANAES recommends the use of the Bethesda system. Moreover, when appropriate, the report must specify why a smear cannot be interpreted.

Women with abnormal smear results are not always followed up correctly. In June 1996, the "Conseil national du cancer" (National Cancer Committee) wrote a report on screening for cervical cancer[4]. It reaffirmed the justification for the "référence médicale opposable" (RMO) (French legislation for controlling health expenses – drugs, medical acts, etc. limited for particular conditions) concerning routine screening. The RMO also specified that a periodic gynaecological examination is necessary and must not be restricted merely to preparing a smear.

---

3. *"Conduite à tenir devant un frottis anormal du col de l'utérus. Le frottis du col de l'utérus"* (Management of women with abnormal cervical smear results. The cervical smear), ANAES Report, January 1998.
4. Conseil national du cancer (National Cancer Committee), Notice No. 3 of 25 June 1996 on the organisation of screening for cancer of the cervix in France.

Part three A few organisational problems in the health system

Organisation of screening for cervical cancer

The National Cancer Committee[5] made proposals for the organisation of cervical cancer screening which is designed to improve the quality of smears and the management of women with abnormal smear results.

The attainment of these objectives will be aided by instigating quality assurance testing for the examinations and developing training programmes for doctors and professionals involved: this should ultimately lead to the accreditation of laboratories participating in the screening programme[5], and raise the question of potential authorisation of the professionals.

This organisation should also contribute to a more equitable distribution of the 6 to 7 million smears carried out every year in France by spacing out the futile smears performed every year, or even every 6 months, for some women, and particularly by increasing the participation of all women. To this end, the National Cancer Committee[5] recommends the use of a health record, as well as better conditions of accessibility.

In addition to improving the distribution of sampling sites so as to ensure geographical accessibility, the required formalities should be simplified and above all the smear and any subsequent additional examinations that may prove necessary should be free. However, the National Health Insurance Agency has yet to set up a system for specifically identifying smears in the nomenclature for medical acts. This identification is essential so that checks can be made to ensure that the recommendations for conducting screening tests are applied.

Lastly, the entire programme must be continuously evaluated and coordinated on a national scale.

Screening for breast cancer

In France, the most frequent cancer in women is breast cancer with an incidence of 58 per 100,000 inhabitants. It is responsible[6] for more than 10,000 deaths annually; the survival rate at 5 years is 71%. The increase in deaths observed between 1980 and 1992 appears to be currently slowing down, and even decreasing among those in the 50-69 age bracket[7]. This slight downturn might be due to recent screening campaigns.

---

5. Comité national du cancer, Reports on screening for cancer in France, 1997.
6. ANDEM, *"Évaluation du Programme national de dépistage systématique du cancer du sein"* (Evaluation of the national programme of systematic screening for breast cancer), March 1997.
7. Mamelle N., Lacour A., Anes A., Bazin B., Chaperon J., et al., "Les expériences de dépistage de masse du cancer du sein par mammographie en France. Un protocole commun d'évaluation" (Experience in mass mammographic screening for breast cancer in France. A common protocol for evaluation), *Rev. Épidém. et Santé Publ.*, 1996, No. 42: 34-49.

The risk factors for breast cancer are not very amenable to primary prevention, and efforts must be directed at early detection (HCSP report to the 1996 National Health Congress).

The value of screening for breast cancer using mammography has been scientifically demonstrated in several randomised trials, especially in the United States, Sweden, Canada and the United Kingdom[8]. According to a meta-analysis of four studies, the Quebec Evaluation Committee for Health Technologies reported a decrease of 35% in mortality at 5 years for all the women screened and 43% among the oldest[9]. Hence, it is certain that this type of screening is valuable, given the incidence of breast cancer and the ability of mammography to detect small tumours at an early stage of the disease.

However, although it has been proved that mortality specifically due to breast cancer has been decreased by screening, no reduction in total mortality has been detected[10], and insufficient scientific data are available concerning the long term effectiveness of screening in terms of quality of life.

In France at the present time, 26 departments have organised screening programmes and these differ substantially in terms of their management, quality control, training and follow-up of women who have been tested. For this reason, a "programme national de dépistage systématique" (PNDS) (national programme for routine screening) of breast cancer was set up and officialised by the decree of 13 May 1994, a National Committee being created to steer the programme with the aim of generalising screening to all French departments. ANDEM (which later became ANAES) published a schedule of conditions for the PNDS in 1996[11] and an evaluation of the PNDS in March 1997[6].

Organised programmes and "spontaneous" screening still coexist in all of these departments, and although it is estimated that 85% of the target population undergoes mammography examinations, only 40% of women are screened as part of the organised programme, while 45% are screened spontaneously[11].

---

8. Scaf-Klomp W., Sanderman R., Van de Wiel HBM., et al., Distressed or relieved? Psychological side effets of breast cancer screening in the Netherlands, *J Epidemiol Community Health*, 1997; 51: 705-710.
9. Conseil d'évaluation des technologies de la santé du Québec (Quebec Evaluation Committee for Health Technologies), *"Dépistage du cancer du sein au Québec. Estimation des coûts et des effets sur la santé"* (Screening for breast cancer in Quebec. Estimated costs and effects on health), Montreal: CETS 1990, November, 13 p.
10. Tabar L., Fagerberg G., Duffy S.W., Day N.E., The Swedish two county trial of mammographic screening for breast cancer. Recent results and calculation of benefit, *J Epidémiol Comm Health* 1989; 43: 107-14.
11. Ministry of Employment and Social Affairs, DGS, Bureau SQ2. National steering committee of the systematic screening programme for breast cancer. Schedule of Conditions, 1996.

In 1993, a report by the "Inspection générale des affaires sociales" (IGAS)[12] (Health and Social Affairs Inspection Bureau) on the feasibility of a national screening campaign for breast cancer had already identified the predictable difficulties of such a programme on a national scale, particularly those related to the legal jurisdictions of the parties involved, which need to be clarified: the regional councils are currently responsible *a priori* for implementing screening. The IGAS also made recommendations concerning the quality of the organisation and the need for permanent financing.

Presently, in spite of the existence of the national programme, there are large differences in the level of programme financing (expressed relative to the target population) from one department to another[6]. Moreover, wide differences have been observed in the application of internal and external quality control concerning the key act in screening, *i.e.* mammography. In particular, the presentation of quality control results for mammograms is very heterogeneous and makes any overall summary impossible. Similarly, there is no quality control of breast cytopathology as recommended in the 1994 HCSP report[13].

Organised and spontaneous screening differ in terms of cost and quality: mammograms recorded for screening purposes outside organised programmes are considered "spontaneous screening". In this case, practitioners are in no way obliged to observe the principles advocated by the organised programme (age, recording, quality control, two independent readings, patient follow-up). It should also be recalled that the radiologist is paid 250 F for mammography performed within the scope of organised screening, whereas the National Health Insurance Agency reimbursement for "diagnostic" mammography performed as spontaneous screening is about 450 F.

Certainly these two types of screening provide good mammographic coverage for the target population, but at a very high cost, and the duality of the system lessens the effectiveness of the programme. The quality of spontaneous and organised screening should be the same, at least for the target age group. In addition, it should be possible to identify screening mammograms using the "Nomenclature Générale des Actes Professionnels" (NGAP) (General Nomenclature for Professional Acts).

In a December 96 scheme, the "Caisse nationale de l'assurance maladie des travailleurs salariés" (CNAMTS) (National Health

---

12. Tcheriatchoukine J., Raymond M., *"Rapport sur la faisabilité d'une campagne nationale de dépistage du cancer du sein"* (Report on the feasibility of a national breast cancer screening campaign), Paris, IGAS, October 1993, 26 p.
13. High Committee on Public Health, Report "Assurance qualité en anatomocytopathologie" (Quality Assurance in cytopathology). Cervical and breast cancers, December 1994, 7 p.

Insurance Agency for Salaried Workers) suggested offering a free screening mammography session to all women aged 50 to 69 once very two years. However, will general practitioners, gynaecologists and radiologists make a clear distinction between mammography for screening and mammography for diagnostic purposes?

A law that would make the quality control of mammograms obligatory seems to be required. A new European directive aimed at the radioprotection of patients that institutes radiological quality control is in the process of validation and ought to be adopted in France before 1 January 1999. It will also be necessary to make quality control of cytopathology results mandatory so as to ensure that screening is efficient.

The ordinances of April 1996 make continuing education obligatory for practitioners. In this context, it would be reasonable for radiologists engaged in screening to hold, for example, a certificate denoting that they had undergone previous training in breast imaging.

The ANDEM report in March 1997 concerning the PNDS evaluation[14] noted that the grounds for routine breast cancer screening had been confirmed for the age groups among which it was performed. This programme must meet the public health objectives that it has set itself. From this point of view, the target rate of coverage for a programme with respect to the population in question (70% according to the WHO) is more of an ethical than a scientific requirement. On the other hand, the quality of screening practices and protocols for the management of positive cases must be rigorously framed.

Prospects

On the basis of both international experience and an evaluation of current practice in France, screening for these two types of female cancer is of indisputable value.

However, the results obtained appear to be less than optimal by comparison with the theoretical results which might have been expected and the actual cost entailed, whether for organised or spontaneous screening.

---

14. ANDEM, *"Évaluation du Programme national de dépistage systématique du cancer du sein"* (Evaluation of the national programme of systematic screening for breast cancer), March 1997.

In general, as emphasised in the National Cancer Committee report[15], since cancer screening is directed at individuals who are ostensibly in good health, the authorities who organise it are implicitly responsible for ensuring its quality and outcome.

In fact, screening poses its own intrinsic "iatrogenic" risks for the individual. Screening produces an appreciable rate of false positives which can cause unjustified anguish, unpleasantness or suffering in the patients concerned, because of the additional examinations that must be undergone.

A special study[16] on the false positives of breast cancer screening showed that, two to six months later, women who had had false positive results did remember the stress they had endured. However, upon analysis, they had not been prey to any specific psychological disturbance compared with women whose results had been negative right from the start.

Potential iatrogenic accidents could place practitioners and organisers in difficult medico-legal situations, and the physician is obliged, particularly in the case of screening, to provide the patient with relevant information. He is responsible for proving that he has fulfilled this obligation.

Other medico-legal aspects create complications in setting up screening programmes, if only because of the name-based files maintained for the purposes of individualised patient monitoring and global evaluation of the programmes (application of the law relating to data processing and basic rights).

The National Cancer Committee has recommended that a specific national schedule of conditions for organised screening should be drawn up (and revised) by a scientific committee, the following points being made clear:
– definition of the programme in keeping with current scientific knowledge,
– coverage of the target population,
– training of the participants in the programme,
– quality assurance and accreditation of structures that perform the examinations,
– running of the programme,
– medical and economic evaluation,
– definition of budgets.

The national programme for breast cancer screening has been in existence since 1994. It has not, however, so far led to any standardisation in practices or delimitation of spontaneous screening, which is in itself a disappointing result.

---

15. Comité national du cancer, Reports on cancer screening in France, 1997.
16. Scaf-Klomp W., Sanderman R., Van de Wiel HBM., *et al.*, Distressed or relieved? Psychological side effetts of breast cancer screening in the Netherlands, *J Epidemiol Community Health*, 1997; 51: 705-710.

From the regulatory viewpoint, the law on decentralisation makes the regional councils responsible for screening. However, the latter are not able to effortlessly organise screening with the required rigour and hence detrimental differences occur in the effective application of national programmes at the departmental level. Additionally, permanent financing can be voted down in annual departmental budgets.

It seems increasingly necessary that the State should introduce regulations specifying the elaboration of screening programmes at the national level and making implementation by the regional councils mandatory, if they retain the responsibility for such implementation. As far as financing is concerned, the CNAMTS should identify the screening acts (smears, mammograms, etc.) using specific key-letters so that methods for the reimbursement of organised and spontaneous screening can become standardised, on condition that the latter complies with the necessary quality criteria.

To be successful, the setting up of this type of organisation needs to see changes in regulations and reimbursement tariffs, increased commitment by professionals to quality procedures, and wider dissemination of information to the general public.

CHAPTER SEVEN

Progress in emergency services

The management of emergencies is a highly charged subject in the organisation of any medical care system. Recent developments have shown that there is increasing interest in optimising this sector in France, as instanced firstly by the various reports coordinated by Prof. A. Steg, and then the successive elaboration of decrees and inclusion of emergencies under the instruments subject to planning by "schémas régionaux d'organisation sanitaire" (SROS) (Regional Health Organisation Schemes).

Although no judgement can be passed on the restructuring which ought to result from putting the latter decrees into effect and the adoption of regional schemes which is now under way, progress already seems to have been made in terms of the provision of medical care and the autonomy of "services d'accueil" (reception services). However, certain recent laws are still not being applied. Moreover, improvements in emergency care cannot be restricted to hospital aspects alone – they require a more comprehensive approach to the medical care system that incorporates regulation of pre-hospitalisation and transportation aspects and subsequent organisation of the hospitals themselves.

At present, there is an annual increase of about 4% in the calls on emergency services[1,2], and about eight million patients per year currently present for emergency treatment throughout France, mostly for conditions which are not very serious[3]. This is justification for due consideration being given to the reasons underlying the demand for emergency attention, and to the appropriate social

---

1. Beecham L., UK emergency services need priority, *BMJ* 1997; 315: 1627.
2. Kouchner B., Press release of 7 March 1998, Ministry of Employment and Solidarity.
3. Unger P.F., "Quels patients doit-on hospitaliser à partir d'un service d'accueil des urgences (SAU)?" (What patients should be hospitalised from an emergency reception service?) *Rean Urg*, 1996; 5 (5): 603-604.

as well as medical means that need to be adopted to meet this demand.

In general, the organisation of emergency services is subject to several, sometimes contradictory, constraints:
– effectively dealing with the most serious emergencies,
– responding to the increasing flow of "perceived" emergencies,
– ensuring optimum geographic and social accessibility.

Consequently, the quality of emergency treatment probably depends as much on ongoing improvements in the emergency services themselves as on the spatial organisation and co-ordination of the various parties involved.

Initially, a description will be given of the important points defined by the decrees. This will be followed by details of an opinion poll conducted among the members of the scientific committee and the evaluation commission of the Francophone Society for Medical Emergencies which provides a more qualitative approach to the implementation of these texts. Finally, the steady increase in demand for emergency services which led to a broadening of the debate concerning its precise role is discussed.

Background

Throughout the slow development of the health system, the appropriate reception of patients has consistently been one of the founding principles of hospital activities[4]. Right from the time when hospitals were first set up, the tasks currently assigned to emergency services had been clearly differentiated, *i.e.* giving first aid, and sorting patients on the basis of their condition.

From the legislative point of view, the first circular of 13 August 1965[5] concerning the organisation of emergency and resuscitation services inside hospitals primarily dealt with the operational procedures in this type of service. However, it was not until the law of 1970 ordering hospital reform that the idea of emergency reception was explicitly imposed and subsequently confirmed by the decree of 14 January 1974[6].

---

4. Imbert J., *"Histoire des hôpitaux en France"* (History of hospitals in France), Paris, Privat, 1982.
5. Circular of 13 August 1965 concerning the directive for organising emergency and resuscitation services in hospitals.
6. Decree No. 74-27 of 14 January 1974 concerning the rules for running general hospitals.

The notions of health co-ordination and organisation first appeared in the circular of 29 January 1975[7] which gave directives concerning access to emergency services and the links which the latter must maintain with other departments so as to ensure that patients were correctly oriented.

The decree of 17 April 1980[8] stipulated that emergency reception units be set up in general and regional hospitals. In 1984, following various claims notably involving disputes among firemen, SAMU ("Service d'Aide Médicale Urgente" or medical emergency service), SMUR and private ambulances, the government requested that the Economic and Social Committee carry out a detailed study of the pre-hospital phase of emergency treatment. On this occasion, the Economic and Social Committee selected Prof. A. Steg as rapporteur. The initial report[9] formed the basis for the law of 6 January 1986[10] relating to emergency medical assistance and health transportation and the accompanying decrees stating measures for enforcement of the law.

In 1987, a report from the "Conférence nationale des présidents de commission médicale d'établissement" (National Congress of Hospital Medical Committee Presidents) on the operation of emergency services led the government once again to request that the Economic and social committee study the hospital phase. Hence, in 1989, still under the leadership of Prof. A. Steg, a second report entitled "L'urgence à l'hôpital" (Hospital emergencies) was drawn up[11,12]. It led to the publication of two circulars concerning the improvement of emergency reception, one dated 15 February 1990[13] and the other 14 May 1991[14]. The latter set out the resources which emergency services ought to have at their disposal and was the source of standards with which the "Service d'accueil et de traitement des urgences" (SATU) (Emergency Reception and Treatment Service), as it has been known since May 1997, must comply.

---

7. Ministerial circular No. 60 of 29 January 1975 concerning the organisation of reception in hospitals, particularly of emergencies.
8. Decree of 17 April 1980.
9. Steg A, "L'urgence médicale" (Medical emergencies), Report of the Economic and Social Committee, Paris, 1984.
10. Law No. 86-11 of 6 January 1986 concerning urgent medical assistance and health transportation. *Journal Officiel* of 7 January 1986, 327-329.
11. Steg A., "L'urgence à l'hôpital" (Hospital emergencies), Report of the Economic and Social Committee, Paris, 1989.
12. Larcan A, "L'accueil des urgences à l'hôpital" (Reception of emergencies in hospital), *Bull Acad Natl Med*, 1991; 175 (3): 363-373.
13. Circular No. DH DGS-90.326 of 15 February 1990 concerning the improvement of emergency reception.
14. Circular No. DH. 4B/DGS 3E/91 of 14 May 1991 concerning the improvement in emergency reception services in general hospitals: guide to organisation.

Even if these reports have been the source of financial actions[15], measures concerning the quality of emergency care and a legal framework, no real restructuring of the emergency services has taken place.

In 1991, following a strike by hospital anaesthetists and resuscitators, the government created the "Commission nationale de restructuration des urgences" (National Commission on Emergency Restructuring), making Prof. A. Steg its chairman. It had two purposes, namely the grouping together of emergency services and the provision of medical care in such services. For this, the Commission used the results form the 1990 national survey carried out in public establishments by the National Health Directorate and, for the first time, suggested restructuring emergency services into two levels: the "services d'accueil des urgences" (SAU) (Emergency Reception Services) and the "antennes d'accueil et d'orientation" (ANACOR) (Reception and Orientation Unit).

The report published in 1993[16] was the precursor of a long phase of preparation for future decrees in 1995, amended in 1997. As well as setting up a procedure for authorisation, its main recommendations concerned the training of personnel belonging to the services, making the services autonomous, reinstating general practitioners in the emergency system, and improving the co-ordination between public and private hospitals[17].

The basic essentials of the report are found in the decree of 9 May 1995[18,19] relating to the technical operating conditions which health care institutions must satisfy in order to be authorised to carry out the activity of emergency reception. No decree stating measures for enforcement was published and hence it could not be implemented.

The last decree of 30 May 1997[20,21] adopted the operating standards previously set out and incorporated the new provisions concerning the edicts of April 1996.

---

15. Steg A., "Les experts médicaux: à propos des rapports sur les urgences" (Medical experts: concerning reports on emergencies). *In:* Durand-Zaleski, I. *Politiques de santé en France: quelle légitimité pour quels décideurs?* Paris, Médecine-Sciences Flammarion, 1997, pp. 17-19.
16. Steg A., "La médicalisation des urgences" (The provision of medical care for emergencies), report of the National Commission on restructuring emergencies, Paris, 1993.
17. Steg A., "La restructuration des urgences: un impératif de sécurité" (Restructuring emergencies: a necessity for the sake of safety), *Bull Acad Nat Med*, 1994; 178 (8): 1475-1492.
18. Decree No. 95-647 of 9 May 95 concerning the reception and treatment of emergencies in health care institutions, *Journal officiel* of 10 May 1995, 27-32.
19. Decree No. 95-648 of 9 May 95 concerning the technical operating conditions that must be met by health care institutions to warrant authorisation for the provision of the medical care activity "Reception and treatment of emergencies". *Journal officiel* of 10 May 1995, 33-37.
20. Decree No. 97-615 of 30 May 1997 concerning the reception and treatment of emergencies in health care institutions, *Journal officiel* of 1 June 1997, 211-6.
21. Decree No. 97-616 of 30 May 1997 concerning the technical operating conditions that must be met by health care institutions to warrant authorisation for the provision of the medical care activity "Reception and treatment of emergencies", *Journal officiel* of 1 June 1997, 217-218.

The decrees of May 1995 and 1997

The first texts on emergency reception and treatment and the technical operating conditions which govern the implementation of this health care activity were published in decree No. 65-647 of 9 May 1995 but saw little application. Most were taken up again in decree No. 97-615 of 30 May 1997 with, however, amendments inherent in the edicts of April 1996, namely the instigation of "changeover contracts" [Article R. 712-9 of decree 97-616 of 30 May 1997] and of the task of inter-regional expert appraisal [Article R. 712-80 of decree 97-615 of 30 May 1997].

The latter decree incorporated the role of the "Agence régionale de l'hospitalisation" (ARH) (Regional Hospitalisation Agency) into the organisation of emergency treatment and developed the idea of a medical care network. Lastly, it provided for the setting up of an "emergency" "schéma régional d'organisation sanitaire" (SROS) (Regional Health Organisation Scheme) [Article 8 of decree 97-615 of 30 May 1997].

Provision was still made for two types of structure: the "service d'accueil et de traitement des urgences" (SATU) (Emergency Reception and Treatment Service) [R. 712-66 decree 95-647 of 9 May 1995] and "l'unité de proximité d'accueil et de traitement des urgences" (UPATU) (Local Emergency Reception and Treatment Unit).

The purpose of these two structures is *"to receive without selection and take care of any person in an emergency situation (including psychiatric), particularly cases involving distress and life-and-death emergencies, 24 hours a day, every day of the year"*, [Article R. 712-68 of decree 95-647 of 9 May 1995].

The operating and technical conditions for the reception and treatment of emergencies are very clearly specified for each type of structure. From this point of view, SATUs are the structures which can receive the most serious medical emergencies and they may only be installed in institutions having the technical equipment and range of medical and surgical specialities defined in the decree.

Physicians who work in such structures must be suitably qualified, *i.e.* have a university degree or one year of professional experience in an emergency service [Articles D. 712-54 and D. 712-62 of decree 95-647of 9 May 1995]. The head of the service must have 2 years of professional experience and a university degree in emergency medicine [Articles D. 712-53 and D. 712-61 of decree 95-647 of 9 May 1995]. Similarly, the decree requires specific emergency training for the paramedical personnel *[Articles D. 712-55 and D. 712-63 of decree 95-647 of 9 May 1995]*.

The new regulations are almost equivalent to those of 1995 as far as operating standards are concerned (resources in terms of personnel and equipment), but they introduce a few changes in the medical and paramedical personnel required in caring for psychiatric patients *[Articles D. 712-65-1, D. 712-65-2, D. 712-65-3 and D. 712-65-4 of decree 96-616 of 30 May 1997]*.

Provision is made for the co-ordination of UPATUs with all health care institutions, whether or not they have emergency medicine facilities, in the form of "changeover contracts" which define the conditions under which the co-ordination must take place *[Article R. 712-69 of decree 97-615 of 30 May 1997]*.

For all types of structure, the transfer of patients with provision of medical care must be made in liaison with centre 15 *[Article R. 712-72 of decree 95-647 of 9 May 1995]*. In this context, the institution seeking to obtain authorisation from the SATU must make a concurrent request to a SMUR, unless adequate services exist in health care institutions close by *[Article R. 712-64 of decree 95-647 of 9 May 1995]*. When the patient's condition does not warrant admission into an institution which provides health care, the SATU or UPATU orients the patient, if necessary, so as to ensure that care is uninterrupted *[Article R. 712-73 of decree 95-647 of 9 May 1995]*.

An "emergency" SROS must be worked out before requests are made for authorisation to open such services. The scheme must suggest a plan for the geographic distribution of the patient reception and treatment sites before 1 January 1999, bearing in mind the existing installations and services, the observed or predictable activity and the region's health and geographic characteristics. It must specify which institutions are likely to request the authorisation of an emergency service and indicate inter-institutional relationships (changeover contracts and networks) *[Article R. 712-83 paragraph 2 of decree 97-615 of 30 May 1997]*. Once the SROS has been drawn up, the institutions wishing to carry out this activity are allowed a 4-month period to formulate their request to the "Agence régionale de l'hospitalisation" (ARH) (Regional Hospitalisation Agency) *[Article 9-1 of decree 96-615 of 30 May 1997]*. The executive commission of the ARH decides whether or not to grant authorisations.

The inter-regional expert appraisal mission may, at the request of the executive commission of the ARH or health care institutions seeking to obtain an authorisation to operate, possibly carry out an on-the-spot examination of the features required in setting up an arrangement of suitable quality *[Articles R. 712-80, R. 712-81 and R. 712-82 of decree 97-615 of 30 May 1997].*

The basic amendments to the present decree concern the implementation of these terms in conformity with the policy recommended by the edicts of April 1996.

Opinion poll among emergency personnel

Method An audit concerning the methods of application of this decree was carried out by telephoning thirty or so people working in emergency services (those in charge, physicians and nursing staff) and belonging to the scientific committee and/or evaluation commission of the "Société francophone des urgences médicales" (Francophone Society for Medical Emergencies).

The guided structure of the telephone interviews was based on ten or so questions. The topics broached during the interviews dealt with the application of the decree in terms of the co-ordination between UPATU and SATU, changeover contracts, training and necessary qualifications, the role of centre 15 and the "disappearance" of the post of reception and orientation nurse. Other topics tackled were the task of the emergency service, changes in recruitment by the services, the annual increase in the number of patients, and the role of physicians in private practice within the framework of a potential network. The conclusion dealt with the main obstacles encountered in the practice of emergency medicine.

Results All those questioned considered that the decree is the tangible outcome of ten years of reflection and indicates the government's intention to specifically organise the handling of emergencies. The emergency services have long been poorly differentiated in health care institutions and hence often ill equipped to operate correctly.

Restructuring of the services into SATUs and UPATUs seems to be relevant but special vigilance is required if it is to be really effective and operational. Thanks to their hospital setting and advanced technical equipment, SATUs can, *a priori*, provide suitable care for every patient, regardless of the gravity of the case. On the other hand, UPATUs are less well equipped and give cause grammed. This has led to a certain lack of understanding among the various parties involved and, for some emergency services, difficulties encountered in placing the patients has increased the time that has to be spent in the emergency service, creating for the doctor administrative chores that could often be avoided. The setting up of short-stay hospitalisation units has improved the system but more thought must be given by all the participants involved – hospital, administrative and medical – so as to solve this problem which adversely affects the quality of patient care.

This task also raises the question of a more global review of health policy. The decree reasserted the uncontrollable nature of the provision of emergency medical care. For the past few years, there has been a constant increase in the number of demands made on emergency services, particularly in urban surroundings. The increase is due to the fact that most patients consult for conditions that could actually be treated on an outpatient basis.

This observation leads to a double paradox, *i.e.* the unjustified management of patients by an "expensive" structure and the clogging up of certain services with a subsequent reduction in the quality of treatment for life-and-death emergencies. In the long term, if this situation continues, additional resources will be necessary to cope with the extra work.

Doctors are almost unanimous in their explanation as to why these changes have taken place. There are economic reasons: the patient presenting at an emergency service pays on the spot only for the "ticket modérateur" (patient's contribution towards cost of medical treatment), whereas a consultation in the doctor's office or at home involves much higher immediate expenditure. Hence, the patient may choose to resort to using hospital services.

At the same time, according to reports by the audited doctors, this phenomenon is accentuated by the increasing number of patients who are socially and economically deprived or vulnerable, particularly in urban areas. However, this type of patient would not account for more than 10% of those concerned. Other types of population, such as immigrants, are unfamiliar with outpatient medicine and have a habit of preferentially consulting hospitals and/or community clinics. For all of them, the absence of any restrictive timetable or need to make an appointment, and rapid access to a full range of technical equipment appear to be the three factors which make the emergency services particularly attractive.

For all the above reasons, more and more people are addressing themselves to emergency services every year even though in most cases the medical problem does not warrant such a costly, efficient environment.

On this topic, Prof. A. Steg, in his 1989 and 1992 reports on emergencies, spoke of the increased so-called "perceived" emergencies, sometimes picturesquely referred to as "bobologie" (bumps and bruises). Everyone disapproves of the use of such terms which they feel denigrate that particular part of their activities, and everyone acknowledges that perceived emergencies are only recognisable *a posteriori*, once the diagnosis has been arrived at. However, it is true that some services appear to have experienced an increase in patient consultations for psychological distress. In addition, conditions which are minor in terms of life-and-death require the presence of technical equipment (*e.g.* traumatology) and therefore warrant a patient resorting to the emergency service.

Meanwhile, general practitioners, particularly those in urban areas, appear to have opted out of emergency medicine and this might be an additional factor contributing to the increasing demand for emergency services. Such abandonment is not necessarily attributable to the doctor himself, but is possibly inherent in the difficulty of treating emergencies specifically in private practice.

Hence, in the more general context of a policy for the management of patients requiring emergency services, political decisions must be made in order to curb the increasing demand on such services which are inappropriate and inflationary from a public health point of view. Several proposals could be put forward, but require a clear preliminary statement by doctors in private practice as to their stance – whether they do or do not wish to care for this type of patient and ultimately belong to a network of emergency medical care.

A few suggestions can be made so as to control the flow of patients and reduce the costs generated by such inappropriate demands. If an organisation involving general practitioners, coordinated with a network for hospital treatment, is not feasible, one solution might be to instigate medical consultations without an appointment inside the institution, close to the emergency service. Two conditions would be essential: a doctor would have to be present for "sorting" patients at admission and he would have to be able to re-orient the patient prior to registration in a department. If general practitioners were to be involved in emergency medicine, two developments would be desirable: the formation of a network of general practitioners and concomitant reimbursement for emergencies, and generalisation of the "tiers payant" system of direct payment by insurers for medical treatment. If a network of doctors were established, they could be on call day and night. One of the current checks on emergency care in private practice is that the doctor is unable to estimate the length of this type of consultation – it is not very rewarding financially and plays havoc with his appointments schedule. A network would give doctors the opportunity of organising themselves so as to provide this service without interference in their daily activities. Generalisation of the system of direct payment by insurers would allow patients easier access to treatment and should be included during the setting up of universal insurance: it could be facilitated by using a "carte sésame vitale" (general emergency card).

At the same time, thought could be given to the need for better education of the general public. Patients would have a more suitable choice if they were informed of the possibilities already afforded by existing medical care structures and the manner in which they are organised and operate. Such information could be given by centre 15 (a single, free telephone number) – this would seem to be the most appropriate source for providing facts within the scope of the emergency medical assistance network. In this case, information aimed at the general public would be limited to advertising the role of centre 15. At the same time, messages delivered by the media concerning health matters (whether diseases or hospitals) should be controlled since they frequently lead to the over-consumption of medical care, of which excessive demands on emergency services are only one aspect.

Conclusion

The most recent regulations not only proposed a reorganisation in emergency services into two types of structure having different levels of treatment but also tended to guarantee a minimum safety and quality level by providing such services with adequate human resources and equipment. In this sense, the text indicates a highly positive evolution in the recognition of emergency services. Now is the time to make sure that the decree is actually applied under satisfactory conditions.

ARHs will play a vital role since they are guarantors of the quality of the future structures and of quality maintenance, thanks to the regular assessments they will make. More than ever before, emergency personnel feels the need to put emergency medicine on a more professional footing which they regard as essential in guaranteeing a high level of care[22].

Finally, above and beyond the strictly regulatory context, the present increase in the number of demands made on the emergency services and in perceived emergencies indicates not only a rec-

---

22. Goldfrank L., Brewer P., Warnod V., From the Happy Visitors! *Rean Urg*, 1997; 6 (5): 659.

ognition of the quality of care provided but also the social and organisational difficulties which impede access to other sectors of the medical care system. From this viewpoint, maintaining and improving the quality of emergency care will be a major determinant of the effectiveness of the French medical care system in its present stage. The reorganisation of reception structures within the framework of the SROSs and the division between SATUs and UPATUs must be worked out with the unwavering perspective of improving access to quality medical care[23]. This implies that a true *citizens' debate* should be opened up concerning the purpose of emergency services and what the general public objectively expects of them.

The debate must extend to giving the public information on the correct use of these services, and on the readjustment of the various sectors involved, *i.e.* private practice and institutions, in liaison with the centres for co-ordination and emergency transportation. In the long run, the introduction of universal national health insurance and generalisation of the system of direct payment by insurers will very likely aid in bringing about this readjustment.

---

23. Steg A., "Urgences hospitalières: problèmes socio-économiques" (Hospital emergencies: socio-economic problems), *Bull Acad Nat Med*, 1991; 175 (3): 421-426.

CHAPTER EIGHT

Policy with regards to dependent elderly persons

Changes in public policies in the medico-social sector will be illustrated by the example of the specific allowance made to dependents. In actual fact, the case of elderly dependent persons provoked much heated public debate and many new developments, but its outcome was unwelcome to both professionals and the population alike. This example also throws light on the conditions to be met for improving public health by means of social policies: it takes time to work out a frame of reference for common action, and it requires resources to significantly cope with problems that affect the entire population.

Acceptance of financial liability for dependents: from plans to the choice of experimentation

Towards a definition of public policy

French policy concerning the elderly is generally considered to have begun with the 1962 Laroque report which went beyond the objective of assisting old people and gave priority to keeping them in their own home. At the time, the aim was to encourage the integration of the elderly – particularly the able-bodied – into their surroundings and avoid isolation. In the 1960s, this led to the slow implementation of a certain number of suggestions formulated in the report: adaptation of housing, organisation of leisure activities, development of domestic help, and also the provision of medical care in housing facilities and the creation of sections for medical treatment.

Two laws in June 1975, one concerning handicapped persons and notably instituting a compensatory allowance for third parties, and the other concerning medico-social institutions, played a paramount role in the acceptance of financial liability for elderly persons in difficulty, even if this was not their initial objective. In 1978, long-stay services and two different price scales were also instituted: the latter consisted of a fixed price for care payable by national health insurance and a fixed price for housing payable by the elderly person (and/or his descendants) or by social assistance. This was the beginning of discussions on dependence and *"persons who have lost the ability to carry out the basic tasks of daily life"*. In 1980, a report by R.-M. Van Lerberghe and S. Paul asked for *"the exact extent of the needs of the dependent elderly"*[1] to be taken into account.

For all that, an appraisal of these various measures drawn up in 1980 in preparation for the VIIIth Plan, summarised in the report "Vieillir demain" ("Growing old in the future"), was fairly negative: inadequate and often second-rate home help services, an almost entire absence of any housing adaptation, unwarranted short-stay hospitalisations, insufficient provision of medical care in social institutions, inadequate long-stay care that gave such institutions the function of "old people's home", and a breakdown and inconsistency in health and social care, etc.

The first junior minister's office responsible for old age pensioners and the elderly was created in 1981. In 1982, the Franceschi circular described the actions to be taken to improve co-ordination and to match requirements with the supply of services by instituting departmental gerontological plans drawn up jointly by the State and regional councils. Four years later, these became departmental schemes for social and medico-social amenities decided on by the regional councils.

However, dependency only became a specific question from 1986 onwards, following the preparation of the report by T. Braun in the name of the National Study Commission on the dependent elderly which set itself the objective of analysing the exact causes of this situation and the unsuitability of subsequent responses. The report then proposed "ensuring the autonomy" of old age pensioners or opening up the right to payment in kind within the framework of a compensatory allowance for a third party.

---

1. Ministry of Health and Social Security, *"Les soins aux personnes âgées"* (Treatment of the elderly), Report of the working party on treatment of the elderly, presented by R.M. Van Lerberghe and S. Paul, 1980.

Successive reports then followed at a rapid pace: in 1989, a report by G. Laroque for the "Inspection générale des affaires sociales" (IGAS) (Health and Social Affairs Inspection Bureau), in 1991, the "Boulard report" by the social affairs commission of the French National Assembly and the "Schopflin report" submitted to the government by a group of experts as part of the Commission's work on the plan; in 1992, the IGAS annual report also mentioned this question and devoted a specific report to it in 1993, again under the responsibility of G. Laroque. Five private Member's bills were formulated meantime between 1991 and 1993 concerning the acceptance of financial liability for dependents with a view to instituting a dependency allowance for the elderly. But none of these plans saw the light of day.

In 1991, B. Jobert qualified this slow process of defining a policy concerning the dependency of the elderly[2] as "exemplary indecisiveness" and put forward the following reasons to explain it. Firstly, the problem of dependency was not sufficiently under the control of the professionals who might have got hold of it so as to increase their influence: measures adopted since the beginning of the 1960s have proved to be effective for helping the elderly with very low incomes and limited handicaps, but they are totally unsuitable for meeting the needs of those who are heavily dependent. Secondly, dependent persons and their families are not an organised social group which could apply pressure on public opinion, unlike those with handicaps.

But the obstacles were also doubtless due to the succession of different governments throughout this period. According to B. Jobert, *"these repeated delays were due to the government's great reluctance to open the sluice gates to a costly policy when the control of public expenditure had been made a key factor in economic strategy... It is politically far easier to reject a novel policy than to get rid of lame duck policies that have already been introduced"* (ibid., p. 51). This was the situation on the eve of the decision to experiment and evaluate a new allowance for a one-year period, before contemplating any generalisation.

The choice of experimentation

Faced with these obstacles, the French chose to promote, by means of on-site experimentation, some of the proposals mentioned in the latest expert reports, as well as the principle of an

---

2. According to Mr. Jobert, it counts as "indecisiveness when public policy is recognised as urgently necessary in political speeches and yet this repeated recognition fails to result in any practical action".
Jobert B., *"Une non-décision exemplaire: les pouvoirs publics et la politique de dépendance des personnes âgées"* (Exemplary indecisiveness: the authorities and policy towards dependency among the elderly) in Kuty O., Legrand S.-M., *Politiques de santé et vieillissement*, AISLF, Universities of Liège and Nancy, 1993, p. 49.

assessment so that nation-wide generalisation could be envisaged. Under heading IV with its miscellaneous provisions, law No. 94-637 of 25 July 1994 concerning social security established the principle of departmental experimentation regarding a dependency allowance paid to elderly dependent persons living in an individual place of residence.

The experiments were initiated on 1 January 1995 in twelve of the departments which volunteered: initially this was for a one-year period, according to the departmental agreements reached between the various parties involved. The schedule of conditions defined all the characteristics of the experiments, serving as a reference for the departments selected, and setting a certain number of objectives:
– to validate a scale for evaluating dependency;
– to provide coordinated information to the elderly and their families concerning available services, help and their orientation;
– to encourage better matching of supply with demand at the departmental level;
– to assess the number of recipients concerned and work out the overall cost of accepting the financial liability for dependency.

The lessons learned from experimentation

Allowance coverage: only a minority, *i.e.* one dependent person out of nine, took advantage[3] of the allowance under the conditions defined by the experimentation[4]. The weak impact of such a policy – universally considered to be top priority – was due to the amount of assistance given by surrounding family members, but the conditions for allocating the allowance also played a role. The visit made to the home of the applicant by the medico-social team in order to evaluate the applicant's needs was viewed by the recipient of the assistance as intimidating, as was the mandatory signing of an assistance contract between the recipient and the institutions, and lastly a ceiling on income restricted assistance to the most destitute.

Use of the AGGIR scale: this proved useful and was easy to apply in measuring dependency.

On the other hand, it was found to be inadequate for implementing the assistance plan.

The departmental technical team, after examining the social dossiers, often recognised as dependent persons in the "moderately

---

3. The number of dependent persons is estimated here using the method suggested by Lebeaupin A. and Nortier F. in "Les personnes âgées dépendantes: situation actuelle et perspectives d'avenir" (Elderly dependent persons: current situation and future prospects). INSEE social data, 1996.
4. Income ceiling of 10,000 F, compliance with the procedure for assessment of dossiers including the medico-social evaluation in the patient's home, but no recuperation by the Regional Councils concerning lineal inheritances (inheritance by children).

Policy with regards to dependent elderly persons

dependent" "groupe isoressource" (isoressource group) (GIR 4) and in 20% of cases persons from the least dependent groups (GIR 5 and 6).

WHAT IS THE AGGIR SCALE?

The AGGIR scale is an instrument used to:
– evaluate the degree of autonomy of an elderly person, thanks to the observation of activities carried out alone, and
– define the required resources as a function of the person's loss of autonomy.
AGGIR is an acronym for "autonomie gérontologique groupes isoressources" (gerontological autonomy isoresource groups).

AGGIR is a summarised version of the most common scales for measuring autonomy and includes 10 discriminant variables and 7 illustrative variables. The first set of variables concerns coherence, orientation, washing, dressing, feeding, excretion, transfers, travelling and communication over a distance. These variables alone are used in defining the "groupes isoressources" (GIR) (issoresource groups). The second set of variables concerns the domestic activities of normal daily living: running the home, cooking, housekeeping, etc.

The variables are rated on a three-point scale: the first corresponds to the case when the person carries out these activities alone, *i.e.* unaided and without stimulation, fully, usually and correctly; the second point applies when the person only partially carries out the activities, and the third when the activities are either not carried out or are carried out incorrectly.

The data are processed by computer software which calculates the GIR: this can range from 1 (the most dependent) to 6 (the least dependent).

The January 1997 law adopted AGGIR as the official instrument for measuring dependency and also fixed the minimum level for obtaining the "prestation spécifique dépendance" (PSD) (specific dependency allowance) at GIR 3: this corresponds to persons who have retained their mental autonomy and partially their motor autonomy, but who need every day, and several times per day, practical assistance in defaecating and urinating so as to maintain hygiene.

Co-operation between the participants at the departmental level was notably strengthened by this new form of social action: partnership among the branches dealing with insurance funds, on-the-spot re-organisation to improve co-ordination of the services, and working out of common rules for selecting applications. The management of this new allowance was so innovative that its effects were felt in other areas, *e.g.* child protection.

The "prestation expérimentale dépendance" (PED) (experimental dependency allowance) reinforced the required quality of service, *via* the assistance contract established on the basis of the elderly person's needs and *via* rivalry among organisations which it allowed in certain regions where a monopoly of services had existed. This last observation suggests that the offer of services should be developed at the level of both the associations and the "Centre communal d'action sociale" (CCAS) (Local centre for social action) so as to make the offer more flexible in terms of its timetable, and at the level of paid assistants by improving their skills and qualifications.

However, the PED was a complex, cumbersome system which could not be extended in its then form without assigning additional resources for its management.

It would therefore have seemed logical in 1996, at the end of the experimental period, to adopt an arrangement similar to that suggested by the experimentation, with additional resources for organising co-ordination centred on the elderly person and raising the income ceiling so as to broaden the circle of recipients to more than 10% of those with severe disabilities. But things did not turn out this way.

The specific allowance: arbitration and repercussions

A story full of sudden new developments

While the results of the experiments were not expected before 1996, in October 1995 the government tabled a bill in the Senate setting up an autonomy allowance for dependent elderly persons [5]. On 9 November 1995, the draft bill came under general discussion but was suddenly suspended due to the announcement on 15 November of measures to reform social protection ("plan Juppé") following a record deficit in 1995 (40 thousand million francs).

Responding to pressure from the regional councils who no longer agreed to pay the compensatory allowance for third parties to the elderly, in July 1996 the senators brought in a private Member's bill *"tending, while waiting for a vote on the law initiating an autonomy allowance for dependent elderly persons, to provide a better answer to the needs of the elderly by establishing a specific dependency allowance"*. It was adopted on 18 December 1996 and published in the *"Journal officiel"* on 25 January 1997.

---

5. Meynadier B., "La loi instituant une prestation spécifique dépendance" (The law instituting a specific dependency allowance), Revue française des affaires sociales, special issue "le vieillissement comme processus" (The ageing process), October 1997.

Points adopted by the legislators

The lawmakers took a decision on one essential point in the debate: does a new branch of social security have to be created to assume financial liability for the risk of dependency? This path was not taken, and management of the dependency allowance was entrusted to the departments.

Several reasons led the legislators to confide control of the new allowance to the departments:
– they are responsible for the management and legal social assistance service among the elderly and handicapped adults;
– they also exercise a traditionally substantial, though optional, social action policy;
– by law, they are empowered to carry out planning (departmental schemes) and to authorise social and medico-social institutions that feed and shelter the elderly. It was therefore logical to entrust them with the management of an allowance designed to help maintain the elderly at home;
– they are organisations with close links to the community.

Another argument worth considering is that acceptance of financial liability for the risk of dependency by insurance techniques would not have allowed the community to maximise the benefits of the allowance according to the degree of dependency. Thus, for a long time the CRAMs gave allowances for home help according to the person's income, distributing the resources in an egalitarian manner, irrespective of the person's degree of dependency. This type of distribution paid little heed to the recipient's needs and demonstrated the weakness of allowing social insurance to control the risk of dependency. In fact, the "prestation spécifique dépendance" (PSD) (specific dependency allowance) was innovative in several very important respects.

The most important was that the regional councils were obliged to reach agreements with social security organisations designed to promote co-ordination of the allowances made to the elderly, thereby establishing the cross-sectional nature of the policy. Secondly, the law imposed an assessment of dependency under the applicant's normal living conditions, using a common tool throughout the country, *i.e.* the AGGIR scale.

A personalised assistance plan comprising the aids and equipment needed to ensure the greatest autonomy was developed. All these measures, once evaluated, make it possible to calculate the total allowance required: thus, assistance depends on the needs recorded, but it also obviously depends on the resources available in the department.

This aid is an allowance assigned to, and hence exclusively spent on, dependent persons and personalised follow-up is recommended.

The law establishing the new allowance must be accompanied by a reform in the fixing of a price scale for institutions accommodating dependent elderly persons. This other aspect of the law which makes provision for a relationship between the degree of dependency and the fixing of the price scale is raising many questions since no decrees have yet been issued stating measures for enforcement of the law.

Initial results from evaluation of the "prestation spécifique dépendance" (PSD) (specific dependency allowance)

The first results concerning the new allowance have brought to light fairly contradictory trends[6].

On the positive side, it is acknowledged that resorting to a multidisciplinary evaluation of needs and an assistance plan allows a dialogue between the social and health aspects and probably a view of all the different links which exist between an individual and the setting in which he lives.

But there are two major limitations to this dialogue:
– the medico-social team which fills out the AGGIR scale and organises the medical care plan is not the team which puts it into practice and this can lead to differences in assessment. It raises the more general question of co-ordination among the various participants, which only becomes a reality after a long period of working together;
– services to the individual financed by the dependency allowance are quite separate from the personal hygiene care provided by nurses. However, nurses or home helps can supply the same medical care to two persons, the distinction being based on the fact that one is reimbursed by national health insurance and the other is not. Thus, those who help in the home are less well qualified and less well paid than nurses and primarily assist poor, dependent recipients of the PSD, while nurses usually assist those persons who are "only" dependent.

At the institutional level, the collaboration between regional councils and social security and retirement funds, which legislators had asked for, is increasingly seen as essential to ensure a consistent public response but is still not very well developed.

Certain practical difficulties have arisen during implementation organised by the various departments, for example: some departments include the value of personal property in calculating income, and this dissuades potential recipients. The image of a policy of support for extreme dependency reserved for the very poorest is ill accepted, since the work load and emotional burden on the families are unrelated to income. Finally, there is keen disappointment among applicants belonging to dependency group

---

6. *La PSD un an après: premières tendances* (The specific dependency allowance one year later: initial trends), Studies carried out by ODAS at the request of the Social Affairs Commission of the Senate, Cahiers de l'ODAS, January 1998.

4 since it corresponds to disability levels that the "Commission technique d'orientation et de reclassement professionnel" (COTOREP) (Technical Commission on Professional Orientation and Reclassification)[7] assigned an allowance in previous years.

The complexity of these choices is doubtless one of the reasons why defining the policy is such a slow process, following on from a series of official reports which all stress the necessity of reforming existing arrangements and the pressing need to reply to the demographic challenges of ageing. Almost twenty years of debating, formulating expert opinions and planning have partly helped to remove ambiguities: a choice has been made in favour of social assistance since dependency is not necessarily a sign of poverty. The selection of an "elderly poor" population is a very serious limitation on the reach of a policy which set out to be exemplary.

In quantitative terms, the new allowance fails to cover the need for assistance of the majority of dependent persons. On the basis of estimates made by A. Lebeaupin and F. Nortier[8], the number of elderly dependent persons must have been 660,000 at the start of the 1990s (including 290,000 confined to bed or an armchair and 370,000 who require the daily help of a third party to get washed and dressed) and about 700,000 in 1995. The number of persons who have taken advantage of the PSD between initial application of the law and March 1998 – and who are still benefiting from it at the present – is 31,700 in 78 departments, *i.e.* approximately 40,700 persons in all the departments. Obviously, the figures are rapidly changing since the load on this arrangement is increasing. It should be recalled that in 1995, SESI[9] estimated that 210,000 persons aged 60 and over were paid a compensatory allowance for third parties. How many people will receive a PSD at the end of the current transitional period? It is impossible to say and this raises a big question mark as to the future of the allowance.

Without an increase in the number of recipients, would there not have been an improvement in the quality of services and hence in the health status of dependent persons?

Has the quality of assistance improved at all?

The PSD is a payment in kind: the amount of the allowance is calculated on the basis of the assistance plan drawn up by the

---
7. Technical Commission on Professional Orientation and Reclassification.
8. Lebeaupin A., Nortier F. *op. cit.*
9. Ministry of Employment and Solidarity, SESI, *Données sur la situation sanitaire et sociale en France*, Paris, La Documentation française, 1998, 246 p.

medico-social team in co-ordination with the elderly person or his/her guardian. The assistance plan takes into account the elderly person's state of dependency as well as his "surroundings".

In the home, the allowance must essentially be used as payment for the home help's work time. The work may be carried out either by an employee hired directly by the elderly person, or by an employee hired through the intermediary of an authorised agency; in either case, the elderly person is the employer. The person may also use a contract organisation, in which case the home help is paid by the organisation.

The PSD may also be used within the framework of a family unit, *i.e.* a private individual who, in return for remuneration, agrees to look after an elderly dependent person in his/her own home.

The elderly person may hire a member of his family, other than his/her spouse or the person with whom he/she co-habits.

According to the law, employees paid to provide domestic assistance to an elderly person allocated a PSD are eligible for training financed by pay deductions, but the practical means of reimbursing such training have yet to be worked out.

Variations in the amount of the PSD in different departments

In a survey covering thirty departments, ODAS[10] showed that the portion allocated to the various categories providing domestic help was decided by the regional councils.

"Twelve departments appear to favour the employment of professionals by fixing one or more rates for contract organisations, one rate for authorised agencies, and the same or a lower rate for employment by mutual agreement".

"Eighteen departments appear to favour the use of the most economical formulae. Thirteen departments only make provision for a single contractual rate (from 40 to 60 francs), described as temporary".

Yet the reference rate used in calculating the allowance exerts the greatest influence on the choice of service: a highly dependent person whose assistance is calculated on the basis of 50 F per hour cannot afford contract organisations which frequently hire qualified personnel and can provide coordinated, continuous service whilst offering better working conditions to their employees.

---

10. *Cahiers de l'ODAS*, op. cit.

Increasing precariousness in the use of home help

Professionals in the home help sector are beginning to see their job take shape around the new requirements of the elderly: the need for personal assistance is gradually being added to the need for help in the house. Since the role of home help is changing, it seemed essential to prepare these professionals for the job of domestic help by providing suitable training for a "certificat d'aptitude aux fonctions d'aide à domicile" (CAFAD) (Certificate of education for those who have received home help training).

This training is given on the job and professionals have often therefore obtained their CAFAD while working for contract organisations and authorised agencies.

Training covers the psychological as well as physical support of dependent persons, and the maintenance of, and respect for, the autonomy of the dependent elderly. During their training, home helps are taught to reflect on their professional practice, and to adopt a detached attitude concerning the effects of their professional behaviour on those being assisted. They are generally trained to work in a team and to co-ordinate their actions with other domestic professionals.

Since regional councils give preference to hiring the least costly professional helpers (mutual agreement) and the law does not impose any conditions regarding their training, qualifications or working conditions, this gives rise to two paradoxes:
– the least rewarded and least qualified personnel work with the most dependent elderly people who require considerable assistance;
– the most dependent elderly people often become employers, for the first time in their lives, of professional helpers.

While the PSD could provide the opportunity for defining a real status for these employees and their working conditions, what is actually happening is that the employment of home help is becoming more precarious. The situation is made worse by the State's disengagement from the financing of CAFAD training.

Co-ordination of services and the parties involved

Considering the amount of the allowance, the most dependent persons make little call on coordinated services. Yet these are the people with the greatest need (physical, psychological and social), who often "demand" a great deal from those involved, and frequently require several categories of professionals (nurses, auxiliary nurses, physiotherapists, etc.) at home.

Several home helps are needed for any given dependent person so as to provide effective support (work on personal independence and autonomy), to ensure continuity in the person's management, and to sustain psychological responsiveness among home helps and avoid professional wear and tear. To ensure that the management programme is consistent, it is vital to co-ordinate the way in which each professional plays his role.

These two conditions can be met if the home helps are employed by a contract organisation.

In conclusion, the ways in which help to dependent persons is managed lead to the selection of the most economical solutions which allow little room for the training and correct co-ordination of professionals. Hence, recent changes in the supply of services do not appear to have entailed any improvement in quality, for want of greater quantity.

CHAPTER NINE

Comments

The three examples given above demonstrate the difficulties encountered in putting a consistent approach to public health into practice. On a broader scale, these analyses impel us to reflect on the efforts which should be made so as to **reduce compartmentalisation** in the health system, **simplify statutory arrangements**, and improve co-ordination among participants and institutions. It will also be a question of **developing the evaluation** of health programmes and reinforcing approaches that ensure better quality in the acts performed and in the **training of professionals**. **Information of the general public** is itself also an important stake if changes affecting the health system are to be successful.

Compartment-alisation in the health system

Compartmentalisation in the health system remains a major problem, even if some improvements have been noted over the last five years, especially with the holding of national and regional health congresses, the launching of regional health programmes, the setting up of Regional Hospitalisation Agencies, Regional Unions of Physicians in Private Practice and URCAMs which group together regional branches of the National Health Insurance Agency throughout the country. At the national level, the laws on financing the social security system have brought the management organisations and political decision makers closer together, since Parliament is now responsible for determining changes in expenditure.

However, the principles of the law on decentralisation, by giving the regions or departments autonomy in handling certain health problems, gradually introduce factors that cause administrative compartmentalisation and difficulties in co-ordinating public health actions nation-wide. Other examples of compartmentalisation also exist, e.g. between institutional partners, regional councils and the National Health Insurance Agency.

Part three A few organisational problems in the health system

The example of screening for female cancers clearly shows the need to invent screening programmes that cover the whole country, comply with scientific recommendations, and set optimum conditions for safety and effectiveness. As we have seen, such a programme exists for breast cancer screening, but none has yet been formally set up for the screening of cervical cancer. In these areas, moreover, the compartmentalisation between screening and medical care is highly artificial, since more than half the mammograms for screening purposes and almost all vaginal smears are performed on outpatients and reimbursed by the National Health Insurance Agency in the same way as other types of medical care.

Regional councils are responsible for screening, which is partially financed by social security. Hence, considerable efforts must be expended to ensure co-ordination, and it seems that the State should assume greater responsibility in this area. It must guarantee the methodology, and the latter must lead to the elaboration of specific schedules of conditions, compliance with which must become obligatory for each department. The State must also retain authority over the application of quality controls and rules of accreditation to be introduced, and must make every effort to see that access is open to all those who might benefit from screening. This assumes that the gap which still persists between medical treatment and preventive medicine can be bridged, particularly in terms of financing.

For the link between medical care and prevention to become more compatible, and in order to simplify reimbursement procedures for both users and health professionals, it is of urgent importance that the National Health Insurance Agency identify the acts performed in screening which comply with approved programmes. Such acts would then be charged by the National Health Insurance Agency to the various relevant budgets or financial structures involved. This would be similar in principle to the "pivotal insurance funds" that exist for hospitals, but would be designed for users in this case.

This idea of a single financial operator should also be developed in the area of assistance to elderly dependent persons. In actual fact, assistance which is considered to replace work provided by the family, *i.e.* normal everyday tasks, other than technical care given by health professionals, falls within the scope of the departments. Under these conditions, the division between health and social aspects has not been modified by the law. Only a policy based on a single method of financing would avoid the endless debate on what counts as technical medical care and what comes under the heading of assistance and social action.

The specific dependency allowance introduces an interesting arrangement for co-ordination by linking up departmental services with those of the State: this is achieved by means of a constitutive agreement of the PSD and by getting professionals from the social and medical sectors to meet together in the elderly person's home so as to work out a plan of assistance.

However, this objective is far from fully attained: the arrangement is clearly steered by the regional council and the State services have taken very little part, given their feeling of exclusion from the new arrangement. In the field, the medico-social assessment which legislators desire is *a priori* a good measure, but it could become counterproductive and create additional formalities if the definition of the assistance plan is worked out in parallel with the co-ordination provided by professionals supplying domestic services or aid associations.

As far as emergencies are concerned, recent texts have introduced the notion of changeover contracts and placed relationships for inter-institutional co-ordination on a formal footing so as to optimise the functioning of local emergency and reception treatment units. Uncertainties remain over the conditions for implementation of these texts in practice. Moreover, this breaking down of compartmentalisation between institutions by forming networks for dealing with emergencies ought to be accompanied by greater co-ordination with centres controlling emergencies prior to hospital admission.

Institutions aside, de-compartmentalisation should go hand in hand with improved co-ordination among those involved. On the one hand, the gradual disengagement of general practitioners from the management of emergencies must be checked; in particular, these professionals should be more strongly urged to respond to requests for intervention by the control centres, the more so since community medicine is involved in the operation and organisation of such centres. On the other hand, the medico-social sector should also be integrated at the level of the emergency reception units, so as to provide the most appropriate response to presenting cases. The application of the law relating to exclusion will probably make emergency reception services even more attractive, since plans have been made for persons who are socially excluded to receive free drugs and medical care in such services.

In terms of financing, the setting up of universal national health insurance coverage should allow the entire population better access to the various methods for reimbursing emergencies. In addition, the access to community medicine could be made easier by generalisation of the system of direct payment by insurers to all practitioners.

Part three — A few organisational problems in the health system

Simplification of statutory arrangements

The simplification of statutory arrangements is an important step to be undertaken by the State, although all too often a new law or new plan of action adds to those already in existence, increasing the complexity of the health system, eroding its efficiency if not its effectiveness.

In the case of the specific dependency allowance, the review of policy towards dependent persons could have been the occasion for carrying out a simplification. Keeping the PSD in the bosom of departmental policies has led to the replacement of a single benefit for the handicapped (ACTP) by two allowances. The benefit has been kept for those under 60 years of age and another allowance under greater control by the departments has been added to it (the PSD). Additionally, during the transitional period between the two arrangements, the scene is even more complicated since the two systems co-exist for those over 60. Finally, we should not forget that the specific dependency allowance is being applied while waiting for an autonomy allowance which might re-appear with the next elections...

Where cancer screening and emergencies are concerned, simplification of the methods for reimbursement and clarification of the responsibilities of the various structures will also improve public access and correct functioning of the programmes.

Progress still needs to be made and will depend both on the State's regulatory actions and on regional or local initiatives involving the institutions or partners.

Evaluation

Concerning evaluation, the High Committee on Public Health stressed in its 1994 report that a positive approach should be more widely adopted in the development of evaluation. The examples analysed show that real progress has been made.

In the case of the elderly, the standardisation introduced by the AGGIR scale in assessing dependency made it easier to carry out national studies, and to draw up comparisons of geographical sectors, and different periods.

Evaluation also forms one of the bases in the construction of national cancer screening programmes. The State must be given all data concerning those who participate in the programmes, the conformity of actions with respect to the anticipated objectives, medical efficacy, and the estimated ensuing costs. The State must make the results public so as to inform professionals and the general public alike.

Among the cases analysed, evaluation of the reception of emergencies is still not fully developed. The activity itself does not come under the PMSI (except for patients who are subsequently hospitalised). This gap might be filled in the future by the scheduled development of an information system for outpatients, but it would appear advisable to have a standardised tool specifically suited to emergencies. It is important to be able to monitor more closely, and on the basis of appropriate information concerning medical care, changes in the demands made on emergency reception services, especially so as to gauge the effect of the new arrangements on the functioning of the entire system.

Training of professionals

The development of training for professionals, whether initial training or continuing education fully suited to both the actual activity and public health objectives to be achieved, is still at an embryonic stage. The High Committee on Public Health has been making this comment regularly for the past six years with very little success in changing the situation.

In screening for cancer, the training of professionals forms an integral part of the quality assurance of such programmes. In fact, regardless of the changes that may be made in the administrative organisation of screening, the crucial point is that an adequate number of competent practitioners must be available, *i.e.* radiologists, pathologists, gynaecologists and general practitioners. Action must be taken not only with regard to the initial teaching programmes in schools of medicine, but also among learned societies and colleges for teachers of the various disciplines, and professional associations.

While there may be enough teachers and sites available for training practitioners, the structures still have to be mobilised and the necessary financial resources found. The State must assert its commitment to training by introducing the appropriate statutory measures. Perhaps we should go so far in some cases as to propose periodic accreditation of professionals for certain acts which would only remain valid if conditions for permanent training and actual practice were met.

Better training of emergency personnel is also desired by the professionals themselves, so that the conditions of training set out in the decrees can be met more effectively. However, continuing education is another requirement, given that professional experience must be kept up in the field. From this point of view, the mobility of some professionals within the medical care system might provide an effective response, and also contribute to de-compartmentalisation of those involved: emergency personnel could be partly mobile inside the network so that they practised regularly in local units as well as in emergency reception and treatment services. This arrangement might entail, for personnel working in a given hospital, only one day per week or per fortnight, which would be devoted to another hospital in the emergency network. Moreover, the public might be appreciative of the fact that the same medical and paramedical personnel work in the emergency centres so that the only actual difference is in the standard of their technical equipment.

Personnel other than emergency personnel might benefit from this type of mobility since it would likely maintain skill levels by providing greater experience. This might especially be true of obstetricians and midwives working in maternity hospitals with few deliveries to perform, or even surgeons and anaesthetists.

In addition, general practitioners who so desired could be encouraged to assume emergency duties periodically. It should also be borne in mind that certain medical specialists, particularly those specialising in emergency medicine, work in a very arduous field and it might potentially be of interest to facilitate more rapid renewal of health professionals practising in such fields, allowing them to take on other positions or other areas of specialisation if they wish to do so. From this viewpoint, the principle of practising throughout an entire career as a medical specialist in one particular field determined for ever by the "concours d'internat" (entrance examination for hospital work) and initial training for the "Diplôme d'Etudes Spécialisées" (DES) (Diploma in Specialised Studies) is a considerable handicap that needs to be overcome.

Within the context of the specific dependency allowance, we have also emphasised the expectations in terms of personnel training and qualifications. In fact, the State has created conditions for the appropriate training of home help personnel by planning a suitable diploma, financed by deductions from pay. Some departments have created a label for services which meet training requirements. But the effects of these efforts are limited by the fact that dependent persons make the final decision in choosing the service provider and their restricted budget often makes them opt for longer hours of service from less qualified personnel. In practice, the factors responsible for quality are easier to identify, but the financial limitation still holds.

Information to users

Information given to users must provide the general public with a better understanding of the way the health system operates as well as the stakes involved in public health, and the role of social organisations in improving its performance. Users must better appreciate the possibilities for gaining access to available medical care and prevention, but must also be aware of the initiatives open to them, and the responsibilities which rest on their shoulders. Political awareness is required, and it is with this in mind that the States General for health were conceived and are scheduled in the next few months.

These thoughts were already touched on in the 1994 HCSP report but still remain relevant for the three areas analysed.

In the case of screening for cancer, participation of the public in screening programmes will be very largely determined by the adequacy of the information given. The information will have to be circulated directly and backed up by health professionals, especially general practitioners, but the latter will themselves need to be well-informed and convinced.

In the case of emergencies, the public is not sufficiently aware of how, by dialling 15, it can take advantage of medical advice and emergency services so that the most appropriate response can be given to any problem.

As far as the dependency allowance is concerned, the methods of allocation are still not well known, and unfortunately it is likely that many potential recipients fail to take the appropriate steps. Moreover, ignorance of the exact regulatory conditions concerning income and property may discourage some applicants – this would explain the considerable number of dossiers that are neglected after the first step has been taken.

Conclusion

CONCLUSION

Health in France counted as an event when it was published by the High Committee on Public Health at the end of its first mandate in 1994. For the first time in France, a report was no longer content merely to draw up a statement on the population's health, but queried the organisation of the health system, defined priorities, and suggested targets to be attained as well as the initiation of a genuine health policy.

The present report concludes the High Committee's second mandate and is also innovative in that it pays particular attention to assessing the ground that has been covered since 1994. An approach on this scale, comparing health objectives and results, has never previously been undertaken in France. The 1998 report is therefore a direct continuation of the 1994 report. It is the High Committee's wish that this type of approach be developed as widely as possible, both regionally and nationally.

For all that, today's established facts are similar to those previously found. Without going back over the facts presented in this report in detail, particularly the conclusions in the second and third parts, it is worthwhile stressing four essential points.

As far as health status is concerned, France is still in a situation where excellent, and sometimes even remarkable, results contrast with what are at least mediocre results by comparison with other similar countries. Although 65-year-old French women as well as French men may have the longest life expectancy among inhabitants of countries in the European Union, as a nation we stand out by having a markedly higher mortality rate among under-65s – particularly those aged between 20 and 40 years – than many other European countries. This difference is largely due to the harmful effects on health of behavioural factors such as smoking, alcohol abuse, risk-taking while driving cars and motor bikes, lack of protection during sexual intercourse, etc. The fight against avoidable under-65 mortality and morbidity is not basically a question of improving the medical care system but rather of changing behaviour patterns which become ingrained by custom and practice, often even before adolescence; this aspect was tackled extensively by the High Committee in its 1997 report on health among the young. While our capacity to assume financial liability for medical care is highly developed (sometimes even over-developed) and uses up a share of the national wealth that ranks among the highest in economically comparable countries, the same is not true of our ability to act in preserving and promoting health before medical care is required: the latter receive little attention and resources, while organisational consistency is still rudimentary. The same type of situation is found with respect to the assistance given to handicapped or dependent persons.

The second point relates to inequalities in health status depending on sex, social category and region: these remain marked and show no tendency to diminish. As indicated in the first part of this document, poverty is increasing among young couples. A large number of people could now find themselves in precarious situations which would have a negative impact on their health, as the High Committee forcefully underlined several months ago in its report on this topic. But once again, the responses made have been primarily "curative". They come into play too late, when their very vulnerability has already placed those in precarious situations at a distance from the health system.

The third observation worth emphasising concerns the system of information. The data used in drawing up this report are practically identical in nature to those used in 1994. Mortality, expressed in overall terms or as a function of cause of death, still forms the foundation. Virtually the same gaps persist where morbidity, determinants of health status and disabilities are concerned. And yet many data have been recorded, particularly in health care institutions, branches of the National Health Insurance Agency and the commissions responsible for handicapped persons. But such information is either fairly inaccessible or accessible only in an unusable form.

Finally, the multiplication in institutional logics, structures and procedures is increasingly paralysing the actions of the parties involved in health, making it difficult to apply any all-encompassing, coherent logic. The compartmentalisation of institutions gives rise to administrative fragmentation – as incomprehensible to the general population (particularly its vulnerable segment) as to the professionals. And yet there is a growing awareness on the part of all concerned that a cross-sectional approach must be made to problems involving both health and social, outpatient and inpatient, public and private aspects. To overcome these rifts, additional arrangements are unceasingly being made so as to link up structures, procedures, financing and the parties concerned. An ever-increasing share of collective energy is thus being devoted to jumping over institutional hurdles

Conclusion

to the detriment of the actions themselves and at the cost of greater wear-and-tear on the professionals involved.

Since 1994, however, many events have contributed to strengthening the public health approach in France. The statement drawn up by the High Committee and its proposals were met with an extensive process of adaptation throughout the country. At the first regional health congresses in 1996, the diagnosis of the situation arrived at in 1994 was presented in each region by one of the members of the High Committee and the priorities suggested in *Health in France* were opened up to debate. In terms of health surveillance and safety, the decision was taken to create or reinforce appropriate structures. The surveillance of, and fight against atmospheric pollution were considerably developed. Actions were undertaken in an attempt to improve co-ordination in screening for certain cancers. Lastly, the reforms adopted in April 1996 provided, for the first time, a legislative framework for the global, systematic consideration of health requirements so that the allocation and distribution of the resources devoted to the medical care system could be decided. Proposals for the criteria and conditions to be applied to this regional distribution were made by the High Committee at the National Health Congress in 1998.

Although this report only takes a brief period into account (less than five years), changes have occurred in various aspects of the population's state of health. Many have been positive, particularly the reduction in avoidable premature mortality which reached between 10 and 20%, depending on the case considered. In contrast, other trends appear to indicate that it will be difficult to achieve several of the targets set by the High Committee in 1994 within the proposed deadlines.

In future years, any improvement in health in France will require great persistence in the approach that has been adopted. We need to rapidly bring about a genuine change in attitudes and practices which will allow strategies for both health care prevention and treatment to come into their own. Professionals, administrative and political decision makers and every individual French person will need to undergo a change in mentality. Such a change will have a profound cultural dimension which is as yet unfathomed. Too few people are familiar with the fundamental aspects of the situation in France, and particularly how it compares with other countries in the European Union. This ignorance often leads to the proposal or recommendation of solutions that are ill-suited to current requirements. Extensive information and ample explanations will be vital pre-requisites before any changes are made in the health system. However, complete success will only be achieved if this effort is accompanied by simplification of institutional arrangements. It would, in fact, be much more efficacious

Conclusion

to get rid of many of their inherent barriers rather than constantly erecting ladders to climb over them. Even if that's easier said than done.

Acknowledgements

The High Committee on Public Health wishes to thank the following

for their Co-operation

l'Agence nationale de recherche sur le sida (ANRS) (National AIDS Research Agency)
la Caisse nationale d'assurance maladie des travailleurs salariés (CNAMTS) (National Health Insurance Agency for Salaried Workers)
le Centre de recherche, d'étude et de documentation en économie de la santé (CREDES) (Centre for Research and Documentation on Health Economics)
le Centre de recherche pour l'étude et l'observation des conditions de vie (CREDOC) (Centre for Research and Surveillance of Standards of Living)
le Centre technique national d'études et de recherches sur les handicaps et les inadaptations (CTNERHI) (National Research Centre on Handicaps and Disablement)
le Comité français d'éducation pour la santé (CFES) (French Committee for Health Education)
le Conseil supérieur de la prévention des risques professionnels (CSPRP) (Higher Council for Professional Risk Prevention)
la direction de l'Action sociale (DAS) (Social Welfare Department)
la direction de la Sécurité sociale (DSS) (Social Security Department)
la direction des Hôpitaux (DH) (Hospital Directorate)
la direction générale de la Santé (DGS) (National Health Directorate)
l'École nationale de la santé publique (ENSP) (National School of Public Health)
la Fédération nationale des observatoires régionaux de la santé (FNORS) (National Federation of Regional Health Surveillance Centres)
l'Institut national de recherche sur les transports et leur sécurité (INRETS) (National Institute for Research on Transport and Safety)
l'Institut national de la santé et de la recherche médicale (INSERM) (National Institute or Health and Medical Research)
l'Institut national de la statistique et des études économiques (INSEE) (National Institute for Economic Studies and Statistics)
l'Observatoire français des drogues et des toxicomanies (OFDT) (French Surveillance Centre for Narcotics, Addictions, and Substance Abuse)
l'Observatoire national interministériel de sécurité routière (ONISR) (National Interministerial Road Safety Surveillance Agency)
l'Observatoire régional de la santé d'Aquitaine (ORSA) (Regional Health Surveillance Centre of Aquitaine)
la Mission interministérielle de lutte contre la drogue et la toxicomanie (MILDT) (Ministerial Task Force on Narcotics, Addictions, and Substance Abuse)
le Réseau national de santé publique (RNSP) (National Public Health Network)
la Société francophone des urgences médicales (Francophone Society for Medical Emergencies)
le Service des statistiques, des études et des systèmes d'information (SESI) (Statistics and Information Systems Department)

Acknowledgements

for their contribution in drafting the report

Stéphanie Antoniotti
Gérard Badeyan
Annick Bounot
Laurent Caussat
Laurence Chérié-Challine
Jean-Claude Désenclos
Christine Duval
André Ernst
Stéphanie Gentile
Marcel Goldberg
Hubert Isnard
Christine Jestin
Éric Jougla
Alain Jourdain

Martine Ledrans
Annette Leclerc
Ludivine Leroi
Claude Martin
Eliane Michel
Françoise Mohaer
Claudine Parayre
Véronique Pellissier
Philippe Quenel
Nicolas Sandret
Jésus Sanchez
Catherine Sermet
Jean-Claude Zerbib

It also wishes to thank

Nathalie Bajos
Béatrice Blondel
Gérard Bréart
René Demeulemeester
Dominique Deugnier
Myriam Dubuc
Fabienne Dubuisson
Dominique de Galard
Jean-Pierre Giordanella
Jean-Claude Henrard
Marie-Pierre Joly
Bernard Laumon
Catherine Lavielle
Véronique Ledoray

Catherine Manuel
Élisabeth Martelli
Martial Mettendorff
Danièle Mischlich
Christophe Paal
Jean Pasturel
Jean-Marie Robine
Olivier Roche
Yves Souteyrand
Carmelita Stoffels
Claude Thiaudière
Jean Viñas
Joëlle Voisin

and the members of the "Société francophone des urgences médicales" (Francophone Society for Medical Emergencies) heard during the survey among casualty departments
B. Bedock, G. Bleichner, A.-M. Bouvier, M. Desquin, L. Divorne, D. Elkharrat, S. Feurstein, J.-P. Fournier, B. Garo, P. Gerbeaux, M. Gobert, P. Jean, G. Jego, J. Koppferschmit, B. Le Chevalier, D. Pateron, P. Pelloux, S. Nicolas, F. Staikowski, M.-D. Touze.

Thanks also to Riama M'Bae and Myrielle Toi
for typing the manuscript.

Abbreviations

ANAES	Agence nationale d'accréditation et d'évaluation en santé (Agency for Health Accreditation and Evaluation)
ANDEM	Agence nationale pour le développement de l'évaluation médicale (National Agency for Medical Evaluation Development)
ARH	Agence régionale de l'hospitalisation (Regional Hospitalisation Agency)
CAT	Centre d'aide par le travail (Disabled Persons Workshops)
CCAS	Centre communal d'action sociale (Local centre for social action)
CCMSA	Caisse centrale de la Mutualité sociale agricole (Central Branch of the Agricultural Employees' Health Insurance Agency)
CNAMTS	Caisse nationale d'assurance maladie des travailleurs salariés (National Health Insurance Agency for Salaried Workers)
CNC	Conseil national du cancer (National Cancer Committee)
CRAM	Caisse régionale d'assurance maladie (Regional Branch of the National Health Insurance Agency)
CREDES	Centre de recherche, d'étude et de documentation en économie de la santé (Centre for Research and Documentation on Health Economics)
CREDOC	Centre de recherche pour l'étude et l'observation des conditions de vie (Centre for Research and Surveillance of Standards of Living)
CTNERHI	Centre technique national d'études et de recherches sur les handicaps et les inadaptations (National Research Centre on Handicaps and Disablement)
CFES	Comité français d'éducation pour la santé (French Committee for Health Education)
CSPRP	Conseil supérieur de la prévention des risques professionnels (Higher Council for Professional Risk Prevention)
DARES	Direction de l'animation, de la recherche, des études et des statistiques (Department of Mobilisation, Research and Statistics)
DAS	Direction de l'Action sociale (Social Welfare Department)
DSS	Direction de la Sécurité sociale (Social Security Department)

Abbreviations

DGS	Direction générale de la Santé (National Health Directorate)
DH	Direction des Hôpitaux (Hospital Directorate)
ENSP	École nationale de la santé publique (National School of Public Health)
FNORS	Fédération nationale des observatoires régionaux de la santé (National Federation of Regional Health Surveillance Centres)
IGAS	Inspection générale des affaires sociales (Health and Social Affairs Inspection Bureau)
INRS	Institut national de recherche et de sécurité pour la prévention des accidents du travail et des maladies professionnelles (National Research and Safety Institute for the Prevention of Occupational Injuries and Diseases)
INRETS	Institut national de recherche sur les transports et leur sécurité (National Institute for Research on Transport and Safety)
INSEE	Institut national de la statistique et des études économiques (National Institute for Economic Studies and Statistics)
INSERM	Institut national de la santé et de la recherche médicale (National Institute for Health and Medical Research)
OCDE	Organisation de coopération et de développement économiques (Organisation for Economic Co-operation and Development)
OMS	Organisation mondiale de la santé (World Health Organisation)
ONISR	Observatoire national interministériel de sécurité routière (National Interministerial Road Safety Surveillance Agency)
OCRTIS	Office central de répression du trafic illicite de stupéfiants (French Narcotics Bureau)
ORS	Observatoire régional de la santé (Regional Health Surveillance Centre)
MILDT	Mission interministérielle de lutte contre la drogue et la toxicomanie (Ministerial Task Force on Narcotics, Addictions, and Substance Abuse)
MSA	Mutualité sociale agricole (Agricultural Employees' Health Insurance Agency)
PED	Prestation expérimentale dépendance (Experimental dependency allowance)
PSD	Prestation spécifique dépendance (Specific dependency allowance)
RNSP	Réseau national de santé publique (National Public Health Network)

Abbreviations

SATU	Service d'accueil et de traitement des urgences (Emergency Reception and Treatment Service)
SESI	Service des statistiques, des études et des systèmes d'information (Statistics and Information Systems Department)
SROS	Schéma régional d'organisation sanitaire (Regional Health Organisation Scheme)
UPATU	Unité de proximité d'accueil et de traitement des urgences (Local Emergency Reception and Treatment Unit)

List of tables

Chapter 1
Demographic, economic and social, political... considerations

1	"Conjoncturel" fertility indicator	16
2	Fertility according to age	16
3	Number of births	17
4	Number of marriages	17
5	Number of deaths	18
6	Life expectancy according to sex and age	19
7	Percentage distribution of population as a function of age	19
8	Percentage growth and its principal components from 1991 to 1997	20
9	1990 to 1996 Labour Market	21
10	Variation in lifestyle disparities	22
11	Percentage of poor households in 1984, 1989 and 1994	23

Chapter 2
Public opinions and perceptions

1	Replies given in 1992 and 1997 to the question: "Do you associate good health with..."	40
2	Replies given in 1992 and 1997 to the question: "Do you think the following problems affect health?"	42
3	Priority to be given by the State to certain population groups in its health policy, answers according to age	43

Chapter 3
Indicators of health status

1	Life expectancy in France at birth and at 60 years (1996, 1991 and 1981) according to sex	49
2	Mortality rate in France in 1996 and variation in mortality rate between 1991 and 1996, according to sex and age	50
3	Number of subjects and percentage of principal diseases involved in mortality, according to sex	52
4	Number of subjects and percentage of principal diseases involved in mortality, according to sex	53
5	Potential years of life lost (from 1 to 64 years) according to the cause of death and sex	54
6	Variation in mortality rate as a function of the principal diseases between 1991 and 1996 and sex	55
7	Excess mortality among men according to age, in 1996 and 1991	56
8	Excess mortality among men as a function of the principal diseases	57
9	Variation in "avoidable" mortality rate between 1991 and 1996	57
10	Excess mortality between extreme regions (1996 and 1991)	60
11	Regions of maximum mortality according to the cause of death (1992-1994) and sex	62

12	Mortality rates standardised by age, French overseas territories, 1995	64
13	Variation in mortality rates standardised by age, French overseas territories, 1990 to 1995	65
14	Life expectancy at birth in various European countries (1996 and 1991)	66
15	Life expectancy at 65 years in various European countries (1995 and 1991)	67
16	Causes of death for which the risk of death in France was more than twice that in England-and-Wales in 1993, as a function of sex and age	69
17	Causes of death for which the risk of death in England-and-Wales was more than twice that in France in 1993, as a function of sex and age	69
18	Weight of various causes that account for the excess premature mortality observed among men in France relative to England-and-Wales in 1993, as a function of age	70
19	Variation in stated morbidity as a function of major pathologies	74
20	Stated morbidity as a function of major pathologies and age, 1992-1995	76
21	Variation in reasons for consulting a doctor in private practice, 1992-1996	78
22	Variation in the number of deaths and mortality rate due to accidents of daily life as a function of age	80
23	Relative risk of being killed or injured in a road accident as a function of age	86
24	Morbidity and mortality due to occupational accidents	87
25	Percentage of foreign employees in the labour force and involved in accidents in 1995	90
26	Gravity indicators for occupational accidents as a function of age in 1995	90
27	Age-adjusted mortality due to ischaemic heart disease in all three Monica regions, data from registers and data from national statistics, as a function of sex	105
28	Age-adjusted incidence of myocardial infarction in all three Monica regions, as a function of whether patient hospitalisation was possible or not	105
29	Characteristics of hospital management of myocardial infarction in the three Monica regions, after adjustment for age and sex	106
30	Variation in the declared prevalence of cardiovascular diseases as a function of the nature of the disease, 1988-1991 to 1992-1995	108
31	Consultation of a doctor in private practice for a cardiovascular disease	109
32	Variation in the different components of infantile mortality between 1970 and 1997 in France	116

	33 Number of handicapped persons employed by firms with at least 20 employees	121
	34 Variation in capacity of disabled persons workshops and sheltered workshops during the period 1983-1995	122
	35 Prevalence of spinal conditions	124
	36 Consultation of a doctor in private practice for a spinal condition	125
	37 Variation in the estimated number of HIV seropositive individuals, in screening tests and in the seropositivity rate in Metropolitan France, Renavi, 1989-1996	129
	38 Prevalence of HBs antigen in various French populations, 1990-1995	134
Chapter 4 The determinants of health status	1 Percentage variation in alcohol consumption among the young from 1991 to 1995	149
	2 Tobacco consumption in the European Union in 1996	156
	3 Number of adolescent smokers as a function of age	159
	4 Number of injunctions and medico-social follow-ups of drug addicts in 1993, 1994 and 1995	172
	5 Accidents involving bodily harm and death	175
	6 Number of speeding offences	176
	7 Percentage of persons wearing seat belts in private vehicles	177
	8 Percentage variation in the frequenting of meeting places	184
	9 Periarticular disorders of the upper limb	197
	10 Estimated number of additional deaths due to lung cancer and mesothelioma up until the age of 80 attributable to "continuous" exposure to asbestos as a function of the level of exposure (f/ml) and sex	204
	11 Comparison of the number of occupational diseases "acknowledged" by the Regional Branches of the National Health Insurance Agency in 1995 and the "expected" number of diseases	207
	12 Comparison of the occupational disease rates acknowledged as asbestos-induced in Germany, Belgium and France	207

List of figures

Chapter 1
Demographic, economic and social, political... considerations

1	Variation in the spread of salaries	22

Chapter 2
Public opinions and perceptions

1	Perception of health status as a function of age	36

Chapter 3
Indicators of health status

1	Variation in mortality rate as a function of sex and age, 1980-1996	51
2	Percentage of principal diseases responsible for mortality as a function of sex and age group in 1996	53
3	Variation in regional comparative mortality rates 1991-1996	61
4	Regional comparative mortality rates in 1995 compared with the national mean	63
5	Variations in the mortality rates of men under 65 in France and England-and-Wales (1980-1993)	71
6	Mortality due to accidents of daily life (all ages)	81
7	Variation in the number of accidents involving bodily harm, killed and injured from 1977 to 1997	83
8	Variation in the number of killed (at 30 days) per million inhabitants	84
9	Mortality due to road accidents (all ages)	84
10	Frequency of occupational accidents	87
11	Gravity index of permanent disabilities	88
12	Mortality due to lung cancer (all ages)	94
13	Mortality due to cancer of the upper airways and digestive tract (all ages)	95
14	Mortality due to breast cancer (50-69 years)	97
15	Mortality due to uterine cancer (all ages)	97
16	Mortality due to colorectal cancer (all ages)	98
17	Mortality due to melanoma (all ages)	100
18	Comparative incidence and mortality due to cancers (except skin cancer) in various countries of the European Union in 1990	101
19	Mortality due to cardiovascular disease in under-75s	103
20	Mortality due to ischaemic heart disease	103
21	Ischaemic heart disease as a function of the region	104
22	Mortality due to cerebrovascular disease	107
23	Cerebrovascular disease as a function of the region	107
24	Mortality due to suicide	112

	25 Variation in infantile mortality rate	115
	26 Perinatal mortality	117
	27 Maternal mortality	118
	28 Number of cases of AIDS per 6-month diagnosis period	126
	29 New cases of AIDS per 6-month diagnosis period as a function of whether patients knew they were seropositive and whether antiretroviral therapy had been prescribed before they developed AIDS	127
	30 Annual number of patients in the Aquitaine region who discovered they were seropositive as a function of their transmission group from 1989 to 1997	129
	31 Variation in the mean number of strains of *N. gonorrhoeae* identified per year per laboratory, Renago from 1986 to 1996	131
	32 Incidence of symptomatic acute hepatitis A and B in France, 1991-1996	133
	33 Variation in declared cases of tuberculosis in Metropolitan France, 1984-1996	138
Chapter 4 **The determinants of health status**	1 Average alcohol consumption by people 15 and over	148
	2 Deaths due to alcoholism (alcoholic psychosis and cirrhosis)	150
	3 Average tobacco consumption by people 15 and over	156
	4 Variation in the proportion of smokers as a function of age	157
	5 Variation in the proportion of smokers as a function of socioprofessional category	158
	6 Variation in the prevalence of smoking among young people aged from 12 to 18	159
	7 Average daily consumption of tobacco per person aged 15 and over compared with changes in its relative cost	162
	8 Interpellations for simple narcotics use or use and dealing in narcotics, as a function of the product involved, 1980-1995	165
	9 Interpellations for simple narcotics use or use and dealing in narcotics, 1972-1997	165
	10 Variation in the annual number of drug addicts seeking admission to specialised treatment centres	166
	11 Variation in the number of heroin users admitted to health and social care structures for the management of heroin addicts	167
	12 Comparative variations in recognised occupational diseases and those shown in tables 8, 25, 42, 45 and 47	206
	13 Variation in the total number of cases of work-related cancer recognised annually in France	209

List of inserts

Chapter 2 **Public opinions and perceptions**	● The importance of how questions are formulated	37
Chapter 3 **Indicatiors of health status**	● Sources of information concerning occupational accidents and problems in declaration ● Estimation of cancer incidence in France ● Registers of myocardial infarction Monica-France network ● The HID (handicaps, incapacités, dépendance) survey	88 92 104 123
Chapter 4 **The determinants of health status**	● The "law concerning the air" ● The Sumer survey ● Changes in the regulations concerning asbestos in France and abroad	193 194 200
Chapter 8 **Policy with regards to dependant elderly persons**	● What is the Aggir scale?	249

List of contents

	Foreword	7
	Introduction	9
Part one **Background to the health situation**	**Chapter 1** **Demographic, economic and social, political... considerations**	**15**
	Demographic changes	15
	● Fertility and the birth rate have been recovering since 1995	15
	● Marriages and divorces are on the increase	17
	● Mortality continues to drop	18
	● For the first time, the proportion of 20-64-year-olds in the population has decreased	19
	Economic and social considerations	20
	● Economic growth has been slow	20
	● Employment is stationary and unemployment rising fast	20
	● Disparities in income have widened slightly since the mid-1980s	22
	● Change in the characteristics of poor households	23
	Political and institutional considerations	24
	● Stricter legislation governing biomedical ethics has been introduced	24
	● A reform in social protection is on the way	25
	● Health safety measures have been restructured	27
	Health on a European scale	29
	● The limited legal and budgetary framework for health questions	29
	● Increasing consideration of the European scale of affairs	30
	● Health and the Treaty of Amsterdam	32
	● The Community and healthcare systems	32
	Chapter 2 **Public opinions and perceptions**	**35**
	● Overall persistently high public satisfaction with health	35
	● Changes over the last decade regarded as very positive, especially by the elderly	37
	● A less optimistic view of future changes in the health status of the population	38
	● An altered perception of what constitutes "good health" since 1992, particulary among management	39
	● Increased perception of social factors as determinants of health status	41
	● Any priority must be given to the destitute	43
	● Poor perception of the region as the site of health policy implementation	44
	● In conclusion, greater receptiveness to public health topics	44

Part two
Changes in health status

Chapter 3
Indicators of health status — 47

General indicators — 48
- Changes in mortality and life expectancy — 48
- Disparities in mortality — 58
- Morbidity — 72

Specific indicators — 79
- Accidents of daily life — 79
- Road accidents — 82
- Accidents in the workplace — 86
- Cancer — 90
- Cardiovascular disease — 102
- Mental health — 110
- The perinatal period and first year of life — 114
- Handicaps and dependency — 120
- Back pain — 124
- Sexually transmitted diseases — 125

Chapter 4
The determinants of health status — 145

Determinants linked to individual behaviour and the social environment — 147
- Alcohol consumption — 147
- Smoking — 154
- Drug addiction — 164
- Road accidents — 175
- Risky sexual behaviour — 180

Determinants related to work and the physical environment — 185
- The population's general environment — 186
- Working environment — 193

Chapter 5
Overview — 211
- General indicators — 211
- Specific indicators — 212
- Deterioring health — 212
- Unchanging health — 213
- Improving health — 214
- Health and the environment — 215
- Poor standards for measuring health — 215

Part three
A few organisational problems in the health system

Chapter 6
Screening for female cancers in France — 221

Screening for cervical cancer — 222
- Quality of smears — 223
- Organisation of screening for cervical cancer — 224

Screening for breast cancer — 224

Prospects — 227

Chapter 7
Progress in emergency services 231
Background 232
The decrees of May 1995 and 1997 235
Opinion poll among emergency personnel 237
Conclusion 242

Chapter 8
Policy with regards to dependent elderly persons 245
Acceptance of financial liability for dependents: from plans to the choice of experimentation 245
- Towards a definition of public policy 245
- The choice of experimentation 247
- The lessons learned from experimentation 248

The specific allowance: arbitration and repercussions 250
- A story full of sudden new developments 250
- Points adopted by the legislators 251
- Initial results from evaluation of the "prestation spécifique dépendance" (PSD) (specific dependency allowance) 252

Has the quality of assistance improved at all? 253
- Variations in the amount of the PSD in different departments 254
- Increasing precariouness in the use of home help 255
- Co-ordination of services and the parties involved 255

Chapter 9
Comments 257
- Compartmentalisation in the health system 257
- Simplification of statutory arrangements 260
- Evaluation 260
- Training of professionals 261
- Information to users 262

Conclusion 265

Acknowledgements 271
Abbreviations 273
List of tables 276
List of figures 281
List of inserts 283
List of contents 285

Achevé d'imprimer par Corlet, Imprimeur, S.A.
14110 Condé-sur-Noireau (France)
N° d'Imprimeur : 37594 - Dépôt légal : mai 1999

Imprimé en U.E.